─HEALTH─
EQUITY

─HEALTH─
EQUITY

A Guide for Clinicians, Medical Educators & Healthcare Organizations

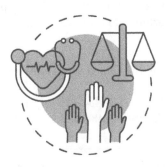

Bonzo K. Reddick, MD, MPH

Foreword by Jarret Patton, MD

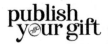

HEALTH EQUITY

Published by Publish Your Gift®
An imprint of Purposely Created Publishing Group, LLC

Specific details of the clinical cases and patient stories described in this book have been presented in a way as to maintain patient privacy and confidentiality. Protected health information has been altered, and some cases actually represent a combination of several patient cases. I want to thank all of my patients for the honor of caring for them and the opportunity to learn with them. Sincerely, Dr. Bonzo

Printed in the United States of America

ISBN: 978-1-64484-616-2 (print)
ISBN: 978-1-64484-617-9 (ebook)

Special discounts are available on bulk quantity purchases by book clubs, associations and special interest groups. For details email: sales@publishyourgift.com or call (888) 949-6228.
For information log on to www.PublishYourGift.com

TABLE OF CONTENTS

FOREWORD

When I first met Dr. Bonzo in real life, it was a splendid day in Savannah. We had lunch and discussed business like old friends. Even though I had met him online a few years previously, that warm February day was memorable for the windshield tour of the town I received after our meeting. During the tour, he enlightened me about the homeless situation in Savannah and talked about the inequities of health suffered by this population.

Through our years working together virtually, I watched him become an internationally recognized speaker and diversity, equity, and inclusion (DEI) expert. After seeing one of his signature lectures, "Why Being Black is More Dangerous Than Smoking," I knew he had a lot to offer healthcare with his expertise. Some say, "it takes one to know one," which is one reason Dr. Bonzo and I hit it off so well. I worked many years as a physician executive for a large hospital system on the east coast. Besides running a medical staff of over 1,500 physicians, I took a heightened interest in health disparities early in my career which led me to complete two different post graduate fellowships: one with the Health Research and Educational Trust (HRET) on cultural competency and the Disparities Leadership Program at Massachusetts General Hospital.

One of my prouder moments was receiving the Edgar Hayhow Award, along with my peers, for article of the year from the American College of Healthcare Executive for "Developing a Culturally Competent Health Network: A Planning Framework and Guide." Although my days as a hospital executive are over, my passion for health equity never ceases.

Dr. Bonzo has written this book from his lens as an award-winning medical educator and an internationally acclaimed DEI expert. By reading this text, you will learn more about health inequities, where they come from, and strategies to improve them. Additionally, you will learn how to teach these topics to our next generation of health professionals. This text should be considered required reading in medical school, nursing school, pharmacy school, and other allied health fields.

After having several visiting professorships at universities from coast to coast, Dr. Bonzo now spreads his messages around DEI to shape the training of faculty, students, and staff. Not only does he teach these subjects to universities in the United States and Canada, but his curriculum also sets the stage for true change in healthcare to make outcomes more equitable across various vulnerable populations.

This book, Dr. Bonzo's first, is set up to change the way people learn about health inequities. Leading by example, Dr. Bonzo not only teaches best practices, but enhances learning points by highlighting bungles—valuable lessons he had to learn along the way. The journey to health equity is a long road that we all must walk. However, Dr. Bonzo demonstrates that we all have our own learning curve that he unselfishly shares with you. To achieve equity, you must be able to examine yourself as part of the solution. If you are on the journey to health equity, this book is a must read as we can all learn from our mistakes.

To improve the health system we all depend on, we all must do our part. The Institute of Medicine has urged us to create a more equitable system since the 2001 release of *Crossing The Quality Chasm: A New Health System for the 21st Century*. This book is one in a tradition of texts to help us all achieve this challenge, not only individually, but collectively.

Enjoy your journey,

Jarret R. Patton, MD, FAAP
Edgar C. Hayhow Award-Winner

PREFACE

SPRING 2020

Several events from 2020 highlighted the inequities that exist in our society in a way that I had not seen in my professional lifetime. The global pandemic caused by SARS-CoV-2 (the coronavirus that causes COVID-19) led to the quarantining of millions of people within their homes at a level not seen in more than a century. These homebound individuals spent a significant amount of time tuning in to news and social media outlets, just at a time when the homicides of Ahmaud Arbery, Breonna Taylor, and George Floyd were making national news. While their deaths had the same emotional impact on me personally as those of other unarmed Black people from the past, there seemed to be more universal outrage over their killings than those of Trayvon Martin, Tamir Rice, and Philando Castile in prior years.

From my viewpoint, it seemed that previously unconvinced people—politicians on television, colleagues at work, parents of my children's friends—were now disgusted by the way Black people are often mistreated in this country. "Black Lives Matter" (BLM) was previously a divisive phrase that some White people were nervous to utter, for fear that they were making a statement that *all* lives did not matter. Now the phrase "Black Lives Matter" was written out in large letters on the basketball courts of the National Basketball Association (NBA) during the playoffs and championship series.[1] BLM became a common hashtag on social media accounts for people from all walks of life.

The same awakening in 2020 that seemed to happen in relation to problems with criminal justice for Black Americans also appeared to occur with regard to health inequities. Early during the COVID-19 pandemic, it became clear that this new strain of coronavirus was disproportionately affecting African Americans and Hispanic/Latino/Latinx Americans.[2] In Chicago, African American people make up 30 percent of the population yet accounted for 50 percent of COVID-19 cases and 70 percent of COVID-19 deaths in one early study.[2]

Similar to national data of predominantly Black counties, this meant that Black Chicagoans were dying at a rate six-times higher than that of Non-Hispanic White communities. In Louisiana, Black people represent 32 percent of the population, yet accounted for more than 70 percent of COVID-19 deaths at one point. In my home state of Georgia, the incidence of COVID-19 in the Black community—approximately 31 percent—almost identically mirrored the Black population in census data. However, African Americans in an early analysis accounted for more than 50 percent of COVID-19 deaths in Georgia.[3] Daily, I heard from physician colleagues who were disturbed that a disease could affect certain groups in such an unequal manner.

PRE-2020

Between 2005 and 2007, I completed graduate school coursework at the University of North Carolina at Chapel Hill (Gillings School of Global Public Health) that resulted in the awarding of an interdisciplinary certificate in health disparities. Much of the academic work for my associated master of public health (MPH) degree focused on the differences in health outcomes for historically excluded groups in the population. The result was that, for the fifteen years immediately prior to the SARS-CoV-2 pandemic, I was aware of what felt like an endless list of health conditions that disproportionately affected minority/minoritized communities. That is why I was surprised that so many other people were surprised about the health disparities associated with COVID-19. These same types of disparities have existed for decades—or even centuries in some cases—for diseases such as hypertension, stroke, chronic kidney disease, and diabetes mellitus.

The Institute of Medicine's (IOM) Committee on Understanding and Eliminating Racial and Ethnic Disparities in Health Care initially convened in 1999, and in 2002 they published "Unequal Treatment: Confronting Racial and Ethnic Disparities in Healthcare."[4] This told us, eighteen years prior to the COVID-19 pandemic, that racial and ethnic minorities receive a lower quality of health care and have overall worse health outcomes compared to majority populations. The source of these differences, or disparities, in health outcomes is multifactorial: an inefficient and fragmented healthcare system, cultural or linguistic barriers to care for immigrant populations, health care provider prejudice and bias—both implicit and explicit—and patient mistrust of a system that has historically exploited and marginalized certain communities.

For the eight years or so prior to 2020, I was a frequent speaker at several national conferences of various academic medicine organizations. My subject matter was typically one of two things: (1) a test-enhanced learning curriculum that I found was one solution to test-taking woes for struggling learners, and (2) health disparities or inequities. The test-taking curriculum that I presented was universally embraced and utilized by dozens of residency programs and medical schools around the country. When I would present on health inequities, however, the reception was not so warm.

Both topics were steeped in evidence and presented with a focus on improving the experience of the target groups—our learners in the case of the test-taking curriculum, and our patients or people in society in the case of the health equity lectures. Nevertheless, my discussions on provider bias, problems with our healthcare system, racism, etc., were sometimes met with arguments, anger, and occasionally early exits by audience participants who had heard enough. I was told by one audience member that racism will never go away if we continue talking about it. Another audience member said that I was trying to train social workers instead of physicians. I was not as frustrated by the response as I was by the fact that the counter arguments were based on people's "gut feelings" as opposed to actual evidence to the contrary of what I was presenting.

MOVING FORWARD

A colleague of mine once joked around that I needed a White person to present my health equity talks for me so that people would listen and not be so defensive. Well, that White person did it on April 7, 2020, in the form of Dr. Anthony Fauci. Dr. Fauci was the director of the National Institute of Allergy and Infectious Diseases for the three decades prior to the COVID-19 pandemic, but he became a household name as one of the leaders of the White House Coronavirus Task Force.

On the aforementioned date, Dr. Fauci said in an interview, "Sometimes when you're in the middle of a crisis, like we are now with the coronavirus, it really does ultimately shine a very bright light on some of the real weaknesses and foibles in our society."[5] He went on to say, "health disparities have always existed for the African American community, but here again with the crisis now, it's shining a bright light on how unacceptable that is. Because yet again, when you have a situation like the coronavirus, they are suffering disproportionately."

Suddenly, in the same manner that we saw in the case of police reform and the killing of unarmed Black people, the 2020 version of America was ready to have a conversation about health inequities. In addition to Dr. Fauci, more and more well-known figures in healthcare circles began to discuss how the unequal treatment of Black and Hispanic people in hospitals around the country is caused by the same forces that led to the killing of George Floyd and Breonna Taylor. The academic affairs deans of medical schools were rushing to add more health equity content to their curriculum. I was now being invited to present all over the country on the same topics that sometimes led to hostility in the previous eight years. Not only that, but people were willing to pay to make it happen. I couldn't believe it but achieving health equity was finally being valued!

HOW TO USE THIS BOOK

Although the global pandemic led to renewed interest in health disparities, I heard from numerous medical schools, residency programs, outpatient clinic systems, and hospital organizations that they did not have the tools to teach about health equity. They have in-house specialists in any field, from cardiology, to pediatrics, to plastic surgery.

They did not, however, have experts with experience in how to reduce health inequities. I decided to write this book as an efficient, multi-purpose tool that could be used in various scenarios regardless of the participants' level of experience. The chapters are not particularly long, which lends itself well to "pre-reading" sections of the book prior to discussions or didactic sessions.

As the name implies, this book is an overview that presents the basic elements of teaching and learning about health equity. It can be used by health educators who teach resident physicians, medical students, or other health professions students. It can also be used by physicians or other health care and allied health professionals who want to reassess their approach to the equitable care of all people. It is written in a somewhat casual manner that explains the basic concepts of health equity in the context of both everyday life and healthcare or health-related settings.

The evidence-based descriptions of the different concepts are accompanied by anecdotes that less experienced teachers may feel free to use to understand and comfortably present these topics to learners. For more experienced teachers who understand the concepts but would like new examples or new teaching ideas, this book provides several cases and scenarios that should help to keep learners engaged. Knowledgeable instructors can also use this book as a refresher to review any of the twelve themes that are presented.

Chapters 2 through 13 focus on specific health disparity concepts, and these chapters are further divided into five sections:

1. Anecdotes and examples of how the chapter's concepts have presented in my everyday life either inside or outside of healthcare settings

2. Examples related to healthcare-associated situations that show how these concepts negatively affect the health of patients and populations. In other words, a description of the major disparities and inequities related to each chapter's main theme

3. Evidence-based methods that can be used to minimize inequities and move us closer towards achieving health equity

4. Using a model based on the IOM quality improvement conceptual approach,[6] presentation of a framework that reviews the *knowledge*, *attitudes*, and *skills*, which can be used to summarize the health equity basics from each chapter

5. A specific case, scenario, shared anecdote, or interactive activity that can be used with learners as an engaging, sometimes even entertaining, example of how to introduce the chapter's premise to audiences at any stage of learning or in any setting.

COMMENT ON INTERSECTIONALITY

Several chapters focus on the inequities that affect specific historically marginalized communities, including women, racial and ethnic minorities, sexual and gender minorities—commonly referred to as the lesbian, gay, bisexual, transgender, and queer/questioning LGBTQ+ community—and people with disabilities. Presenting these issues separately may create the illusion that they occur within a vacuum, but the life experience of most people represents a convergence of several of these issues. For example, the health outcomes of Black, disabled lesbian women living in rural communities will be influenced by the totality of the themes discussed in Chapter 3 (racism), Chapter 5 (sexism), Chapter 6 (LGBTQ+ health disparities), and Chapter 12 (rural health disparities), often in a non-uniform or unpredictable manner.

While this book assists educators in focusing on any one of its themes at a time—to dissect the nuances of each issue—patients in real life will not have just one type of barrier to optimal health. These matters are at times presented here as individual issues for the sake of being able to examine the differences and distinctions of each issue, but in real life, every chapter from this book comes together in a unique and diverse way for each person to shape the experiences of people in this country.

The first chapter of this book further explores this concept of "intersectionality," so that the reader will be mindful that any chapter's topic will come together with the topics from other chapters to affect a person's outcomes. As the book progresses, the reader will notice an increasing focus on how these issues intersect in most situations. At the same time, while best used in its entirety, the individual chapters are presented in a way that they can be used independently to learn the basics of any of the core concepts of the book.

CHAPTER 1

INTRODUCTION TO HEALTH EQUITY
AND HEALTH DISPARITIES

DEFINITIONS

Upon beginning any discussions—didactic or otherwise—of health equity, it is critical to clarify terminology and definitions for several reasons. Complex topics are often defined in different ways by different people, and provocative topics such as the ones included in this book are particularly vulnerable to emotion entering the discussion. This often results in unnecessary arguments based on ideas that are not even being presented. One personal example that comes to mind is from a few years ago when I was listening to a discussion about implicit bias among police officers. A fellow listener became upset at the implication that police officers are uniformly racist, and an argument predictably ensued. Implicit bias and racism are not the same thing, as we will discuss in Chapters 2 and 3, and conflating the two was counterproductive to the intended discussion on how to improve the criminal justice system in our country.

Each chapter in this book goes into detail about definitions for the themes being presented with the hopes of avoiding these types of straw man and non sequitur arguments. Before that, however, we first need to define the main theme of this entire book. What exactly is this increasingly popular idea of "health equity," and how does it differ from the previous buzzwords "health disparities?" This book uses definitions of health disparities and health equity as follows, based on the Healthy People 2020 initiative:[1,2]

- *Health disparities* are particular differences in health outcomes that are systematically associated with, and adversely affect, specific groups of people.
- *Health equity* is defined as "the attainment of the highest level of health for all people," and it is often linked to the elimination of health disparities as a way of achieving this goal.

- The phrase *health inequity* is often used to highlight health disparities that are linked to systematic discrimination or exclusion due to societal obstacles. Health disparities are differences, while health inequities are inexcusable differences. Health inequities often highlight death, disability, disease incidence and prevalence, and morbidity that are preventable or premature.

The existence and origin of differences between groups—i.e., "disparities"—is often multifactorial, and some of the common influences described by Healthy People 2020 include: access to nutritious food, safe housing, high-quality education, and access to health care with culturally sensitive health care providers. Physical and social environments contribute to these health disparities, including the conditions that people are born into, where they grow up, and where they work.

TARGET GROUPS

Given the vast differences between groups of people, there is an endless possibility of disparities that can exist; but there are specific groups that have historically been more vulnerable to social, economic, and environmental disadvantages. Similar to the themes presented in this book, the Centers for Disease Control and Prevention (CDC) and Healthy People 2020 have focused on health disparities that affect specific groups who are demographically identified based on race and ethnicity, gender, sexual identity and orientation, disability status or special health care needs, and geographic location (rural and urban). This does not mean that groups not highlighted in this book or in CDC reports are not important, or that they do not face significant inequities. The framework presented in this book and the foundation that it constructs can be used to reduce disparities and achieve health equity in multiple settings and for multiple groups of people.

INTERSECTIONALITY

As discussed in the Preface, the concept of *intersectionality*—developed by Kimberlé Crenshaw[3]—is important in discussing health disparities, as people may be members of several of the different target groups described above. The life experience of individual people is often the confluence of being a part of these multiple groups, and each person is unique in how this "coming together" shapes their life. If they are subjected to discrimination based on one aspect of their identity, then they might respond by becoming a proud activist for community members who share that identity; conversely, some people respond to these traumatic events by attempting to avoid future discrimination through concealing or suppressing that component of their identity—either consciously or subconsciously.

Each person is different in how they respond to their life experiences, in the same way that our bodies respond differently to similar medical events. Early experiences with families and loved ones who embrace, celebrate, or highlight specific aspects of one's culture cause some people to connect deeply with that identity. There are people, however, who desire to forge an identity separate from their families, so they might embrace other aspects of their intersectional being.

The different elements of a person's identity that are emphasized by that individual often change based on the stage of life they are in, but they may also change from moment to moment based on the immediate physical or social environment. If I am in a room full of single people who do not have children, then my identity as a married father of three children might be more prominent than usual.

As a physician in the United States—where only about 5 percent of doctors are Black—it has been noticeable for most of my career that I am one of the few Black people in my various hospital and academic departments (and sometimes the only one). In these settings, discussions of race almost always involve me, and my identity as a Black man is obvious. If I am in a room full of physicians from various specialties, then my experience as a family physician might shape discussions and interactions. In the days after the recent World Series victory by the Atlanta Braves baseball team, I was frequently seen identifying on social media as a proud Georgian.

Although this description of intersectionality focuses on the perspective of the affected individual, society often dictates the conditions that mold the identities of individual people. Sometimes society even chooses to place people into groups, even if those people do not consider themselves to be a part of that group. Even if I did not identify strongly as a Black man, I cannot control the assumptions that people have about me based on my obvious dark brown skin. I have met people from the Dominican Republic who have the same skin color that I do, but they identify as either Hispanic or Dominican—not Black; however, they would probably be identified as Black by other people if they came to the United States.

For people from the rural South who desire to move to a large, urban city and leave behind their original geographic identity, they may have difficulty doing so if they have an obvious Southern drawl in their speech pattern. This also highlights the point that inclusion in some of the target groups that this book focuses on are fluid and change over time, or they are less obvious at times. Attachment to other target groups is permanent, more obvious, or continuously highlighted in society. Think about the fact that any crime suspect is typically identified by their age, gender, and race.

One final thought on intersectionality is that people are not obligated to "choose" which group they most strongly identify with. The various pieces of their identity intersect to form who they are as a person, and each piece plays a critical part. I do not have to choose if I am more "Black," than "man," although my surroundings and society may dictate that at certain times. Also, if I strongly identify with a specific demographic, there is no standard of behavior that I must adhere to in order to qualify as a member of that group. We will explore this further in Chapters 2, 3, and 8 when we discuss stereotyping.

EXAMPLES (HEALTH DISPARITIES)

Balancing the concepts of higher risk demographic target groups and intersectionality demonstrates the challenges in discussing health disparities at the individual level. That is why it is again important to highlight that this book presents the target groups individually, but an individual's experience is going to be represented by a unique overlap of these groups. The target groups overlap at various levels and intensities, in various ways, and at various times depending on the biopsychosocial environment of the individual at the time. Like in this book, various joint committees that evaluate health disparities have also identified disparities based on individual target groups while acknowledging disparities that also exist for members of multiple groups.[4,5] Take the example presented below of a joint committee that described health disparities that affect populations across multiple dimensions.

The Committee on Community-Based Solutions to Promote Health Equity in the United States—referred in this chapter hereafter as The Committee—addressed health inequities in several distinct populations in the "State of Health Disparities in the United States" chapter of their report.[6] *Racial and ethnic minorities* experience higher rates of chronic disease, but specific minority groups do not see the same distribution of health disparities. While Black and Hispanic people both experience high rates of obesity and other cardiovascular risk factors, Black communities in the United States have high rates of premature death from heart disease, stroke, and cancer, while some segments of the Hispanic community who have recently immigrated to the country paradoxically experience better health outcomes.

In addition to high rates of HIV-related morbidity and mortality, as well as homicide-related deaths, African American people encounter high rates of preterm birth compared to other racial groups; conversely, Asian American/Pacific Islander people have some of the lowest rates of preterm birth. The experience of Native Americans parallels that of Black Americans, as they have higher overall mortality and a large burden of suffering from chronic diseases, however they have overall lower rates of cancer compared to other racial and ethnic groups. In Chapter 4, we will review racial trends in chronic diseases while also discussing the limitations of how racial and ethnic categorizations are used in today's society.

Gender health disparities may seem to favor women,[§] as they have a life expectancy that is approximately five years longer than that of men. However, the gap between women and men has been narrowing recently, and White women in particular have seen an "unprecedented" increase in death rates related to opioid overdose, suicide, and smoking-related diseases. Also, several metrics point towards increased morbidity and a lower quality of life for women compared to men. One example is that women are disproportionately affected by intimate partner violence and serious mental health problems, including depression and anxiety.

The Committee described significant *health disparities for lesbian, gay, bisexual, transgender, and queer/questioning (LGBTQ+) people,* complicated by stigma, social discrimination, and a lack of visibility for people in the affected communities. They are more likely to experience poverty, food insecurity, and homelessness. They also have higher rates of social isolation and suicide-related death, along with disproportionately higher rates of HIV and other sexually transmitted infections (STIs). Although often lumped together by the acronym LGBTQ+, sexual and gender minorities are an extremely heterogeneous group, and even the groups represented by the specific letters of the acronym are very diverse.

As mentioned in our previous discussions of intersectionality, gay and lesbian people do not have the same experiences, but rather each person's experience and their health outcomes will also be influenced by their race, geographic location, disability status, etc. Nevertheless, there are some general issues that tend to notably affect people from various gender and sexual minority groups, so we will discuss an approach to promoting health equity for these communities in Chapter 6.

Military Veterans are at increased risk of behavioral and mental health disorders like those seen in many sexual and gender minority communities, including increased rates of depression and suicide. Both groups experience higher rates of homelessness compared to the general population, and their increased rates of being physically or sexually assaulted can result in long-lasting psychological trauma. Military Veterans who experience combat-related injuries might also have to live with physical injuries and disabilities that can affect their cognitive function, ability to exercise, or capacity to maintain regular employment. *People living with disabilities,* whether military Veterans or not, are four times more likely to report being in fair or poor health. They have higher rates of physical inactivity and smoking, which likely contributes to their higher rates of, and morbidity from, chronic diseases. In addition, disabled people are less likely to receive recommended, age-appropriate preventive services, and they are more likely to avoid medical care secondary to financial barriers.

Finally, the Committee described *health disparities based on geographic location* that exist for both rural and urban places. Both settings have "higher rates of adverse health outcomes" compared to suburban areas, but each has unique characteristics that impact the health of its inhabitants. For example, urban areas tend to have higher rates of violence and homicide, while rural areas have the highest rates of premature death related to chronic diseases and health behavior-related conditions. Residents of both urban and rural areas often have challenges in accessing healthy food options or high-quality health care for different reasons, but the geographic isolation of rural communities and lack of technological infrastructure highlights the need for a special approach in addressing rural health disparities. The unique challenges of rural populations are explored in Chapter 12.

These are but a few of the health disparities that are prominent in this country, and we will explore most of them—along with several others—throughout this book. It cannot be said enough times that the challenges that these groups face do not occur in a void, but they often coexist. While you read about specific problems facing residents of rural areas, for example, think about the other target groups discussed in the previous chapters and how their particular barriers might overlap or intersect if they were also living in geographically isolated areas. Also, look for the common themes that exist from chapter to chapter, as this framework can be applied to the disparities and inequities experienced by groups not mentioned in this book.

INTENT OFTEN DOESN'T MATTER

A focus on achieving health equity does not clarify whether the health disparities being addressed are caused by intentional or unintentional behaviors, or whether they are the results of systems within our country. In my experience, this is a critical point to understand because, as alluded to in the Preface, many of my early discussions on health equity in past years were met with defensive responses. Discussions on systemic racism were often met with proclamations from audience participants that they are not racist and not responsible for racism, so they do not understand why they are being forced to discuss it. For any of the target groups, achieving health equity is not an optional goal that is only dependent on whether the stakeholders capable of eliminating any inequities are responsible for them or not. It also does not matter if the origin of the disparity is nefarious or not, as the outcome does not depend on the intent.

When we discuss in Chapter 6 how assumptions about some women in the LGBTQ+ community lead to decreased rates of cervical cancer screening, you will see that this is often _not_ based on whether individual providers are homophobic or explicitly biased against sexual and gender minorities. Discussions about the motives or intentions of individual health care providers frequently distract from the bigger issues and get in the way of exploring how to construct safety nets in our healthcare system that can overcome our individual actions. The goal should be to make system changes that will overcome individual behaviors, as opposed to only addressing the individual behaviors. We will discuss how to overcome instances of overt discrimination, so I am not minimizing the impact that these instances have on creating health inequities; I simply want to point out that our goal is to eliminate health disparities regardless of their origin.

Here is a simple analogy to drive home the final point of this chapter. Let us pretend that there is water spilled on the floor at your job, and your supervisor asks you to clean it up so that no one slips, falls, and becomes injured. It does not promote safety in the workplace for you to say, "I didn't spill the water, so why do I have to clean it up?" Also, it would be bizarre to respond to your supervisor's request by responding, "You're implying that I hate people in the building and that I want them to be injured. I don't think I've ever spilled water at work in my life, and if I did, I would definitely have cleaned it up, so I don't know why we are even discussing this."

If we apply our emerging framework for health equity to this example, we want to do multiple things: clean up any water spills, develop a system for identifying and rapidly cleaning up future water spills, identify the root causes of water spills in our building, use our system to correct and prevent behaviors that lead to water spills, and find a way to weed out the rare person who purposefully spills water. Asking members of our healthcare system to address disparities of a particular target group does not imply culpability or immoral character on their part.

§*Please see footnote in Notes for comment regarding clarification of terminology used to describe sex and gender*

CHAPTER 2

IMPLICIT (UNCONSCIOUS) BIAS

During the monthly health equity curriculum that I created for our medical students and the one I created for our resident physicians—which both follow the same outline as this book—I always present a bungle of the month, in which I describe a time that I made an embarrassing or clumsy mistake related to a health equity theme. The reason for this is twofold.

First, presenting these blunders in a self-deprecating manner helps to lighten the mood and break down the tension that naturally forms when discussing provocative topics. Although I would argue that these topics should not be controversial, I learned early on that discussing them was clearly divisive to some people and often met with contention (see the Preface for more details on this). Participants in my discussions sometimes think that I am there to lecture them about what awful people they are and to preach to them that they should be more like me. This admission of my botched attempts at being a grandmaster of health equity quickly disavows them of that idea.

The second reason that I reveal my gaffes is that it demonstrates that we are always learning, no one is perfect, and even the so-called "expert" who is brought in to discuss these themes has a misstep from time to time. When leading with errors that I have made in the past, I have noticed that the audience is more open to asking questions or participating in the discussion, they have less fear of being criticized by the speaker or other audience participants, and they are also less fearful of saying something embarrassing since I have already had the honor of being the first to do so.

Each chapter of this book will start out with a bungle of the month that I have shared with my residents, medical students, and some of the other audience participants with whom I have had the pleasure of discussing health equity over the years. For anecdotes that include clinical interactions, I have altered some details of the associated protected health information (PHI) to safeguard patient privacy.

For *my first bungle*, you must consider my background serving as a medical school associate dean for diversity, equity, and inclusion for six years. One of my responsibilities was to increase the diversity of our student body—and thus the future physician workforce—through the recruitment of students from underrepresented backgrounds. The report from the Association of American Medical Colleges (AAMC)[1] describing that there were more Black men in medical school in 1978 than there were in 2015 energized me to engage young African American men and tell them about the joys of health careers and the need for more Black physicians.

Along with this came a need to encourage academic excellence in science, technology, engineering, and math (STEM) so that our young Black students would be competitive enough for medical school when the time came to apply. I was therefore cognizant of the disparities in academic achievement that exist in Black communities, particularly in urban areas.[2] I was involved in several pipeline programs for underrepresented racial and ethnic minority (URM) students to increase excitement about and chances of success related to careers in the health professions.

Fast forward to an outpatient clinical encounter with a young, Black male who was preoccupied with a mobile electronic device and appeared to be uninterested in what I had to say to his parents. He appeared to be in excellent health and had no remarkable past medical history or abnormal objective findings on physical examination. As a result, the visit sped by, and I decided to spend the remaining available time focusing on his social history. I began to discuss the American Academy of Pediatrics (AAP) guidelines on limiting screen time for young children and adolescents,[3,4] which seemed to really pique the interest of the parents—much to the chagrin of my young patient, who was suddenly interested in our conversation. The parents confirmed the AAP's screen time recommendations with me, and they quickly agreed that their son would have to cut back on his time spent gaming.

I realized that I was losing rapport with the youngster, so I asked him what he wanted to be when he grows up. When he discussed careers in engineering or computer science, I explained to him how hours spent playing games or using mobile devices distracts from schoolwork, and that it was important to prioritize academic achievement so that he would have a chance in these STEM fields. To that he replied, "But I already make straight A's." My awkward response of, "Oh! That's great," was paired with regret for not asking how he was doing in school prior to launching into my diatribe—a diatribe that was clearly based on the assumption that this young, Black male was either an average student or struggling academically.

A feeling came over me as I realized that I had somehow formed an opinion in my head that he was not doing well and that he did not prioritize his schoolwork. His parents enlightened me and discussed that he was always one of the highest achieving students in his class.

Somehow this awkward moment had not taught me a lesson, as I was still convinced that I needed to help him in some way before moving on to my next patient; as a result, the encounter became even more awkward. I still must have felt the need to teach my young patient something before leaving, as I began to explore entertainment options for him other than the video game that he had been playing up until our screen time discussion. I recommended that he consider learning computer coding, and I attempted to sound informed as I tried to sell him on the idea of *making* video games, as opposed to just *playing* them.

My young acquaintance educated me on the fact that he was already coding on a regular basis, and his parents concurred that this was one of his favorite pastimes. Undeterred, my pride convinced me that I could still help him, so I recommended specific online coding programs that my son and niece had both used. To that he was incredulous as he rolled his eyes and told me, "Sir, I did that when I was six years old; that's for babies!" It turns out that he was already doing advanced coding programs that were typically recommended for kids several years older. My embarrassment had reached a peak that could not be surpassed, so I congratulated him and his parents for his success, quickly ended the encounter, and moved on to the next patient.

So, what was it about this child that made me assume things about his academic achievement or lack thereof? Was it the fact that he was a Black male, superimposed on my aforementioned interest in increasing Black male achievement in STEM and health careers? Or was it a generational bias that I have, whereby I still have not gotten used to my children who send text messages to people who are physically in the same room, or to my students in class who regularly divert their eyes towards their ubiquitous smart phones instead of towards my slide shows.

Regardless of the origin, I clearly made assumptions about my patient that I was not aware of; had he not corrected me, I might have never realized what I had done. Potentially worse, if he had not been quite the high achiever that he turned out to be, I would have quite possibly left the encounter subconsciously patting myself on the back for helping to plant a seed of success with another Black youth. These are the types of unconscious, or *implicit*, behaviors that we will explore in this chapter.

In reflecting on this encounter, I concluded that my assumptions were based on my feelings about younger generations and electronic devices, as well as my knowledge of reported racial achievement gaps in education. These subconscious thoughts were amplified by my desire to increase academic success in Black youths, which sounds like a noble intention on the surface. However, I assumed several things about my patient without any objective information, a behavior that interfered with a chance to build rapport with him. There was not likely a risk of any long-term harm from this visit alone, but assumptions that someone is not a high achiever could cause harm if they occur in other settings like a job interview, for example. Also, recurrent interactions like this could have a cumulative negative effect on this patient over time.

DEFINITIONS AND TERMINOLOGY

Implicit bias, also known as unconscious bias, is an unconscious preference for or against a particular group of people.[5] Some of these biases develop from our past experiences with people from this group, while some of them grow based on a lack of regular interactions with members of the group. For example, positive experiences with a cultural group may lead to a preference to surround yourself with that group; conversely, negative experiences may create discomfort when you are around people from that cultural group, even if you do not realize why. If a person has not had many experiences—good or bad—with a group, then their biases, opinions, and actions are often influenced by their parents, other family members, friends, and media representations of that group.

In the case of implicit bias, we are not consciously aware of our preferences, so they often manifest with seemingly benign thoughts such as, *I'm not sure why, but I really like him* or *My gut feeling is that she won't fit in around here.* When our attitudes and beliefs are brought to the conscious level, then our brain has the opportunity to either discard our preconceived notions or adopt them as acceptable truths. If we continue to deliberately form these ideas and beliefs, then they become *explicit biases.*[6] The assumption I made about my patient above was initially unconscious, but my conscious brain quickly recognized it once the encounter became awkward and I had time to reflect on it.

To eliminate this bias, I had to recognize that I had adopted a *stereotype* of Black males as academic underachievers, even though I happen to be a Black man myself. I had also labeled a young person using an electronic device as not being serious about school, assuming that he spent all day on his device just because I saw him in one small window of time using it.

Stereotypes are oversimplified thoughts, assumptions, or generalizations about a group of people, without considering whether those attributes fit individual members of that group.[7] Stereotypes sometimes include attributed behaviors or skills that are viewed favorably by society—sometimes known as "positive" stereotypes—but they may also include prejudiced attitudes. *Prejudice* specifically refers to "negative" stereotypes that presume objectionable or undesirable qualities by members of a group accompanied by aversive or hostile attitudes. Although the very definition of the word prejudice demonstrates the harm associated with the thoughts and attitudes of the person holding the negative stereotype, so-called positive stereotypes also have the potential to cause harm, as we will discuss further in Chapter 8.

Discussions of implicit bias often center around race and ethnicity and, as a result, unconscious bias is often incorrectly conflated with racism. Although people may hold implicit biases for or against certain racial and ethnic groups, they may also be biased against people based on their geographic location, gender identity, immigration status, or career. The same way that the intersectional nature of human beings influences their identity and experiences, biases may exist for or against people who represent combinations of the various target groups. For example, an individual might not be biased for or against men in general, but they could still have a preference for or against gay men. As discussed at the end of Chapter 1, the intent of the biased individual does not matter, as the outcomes are often the same.

IMPLICIT BIAS IN HEALTHCARE

In healthcare settings, implicit bias may influence diagnostic and treatment decisions based on assumptions about a patient.[8] For example, if a clinician assumes that a patient of a certain demographic would have difficulty affording an expensive treatment modality, they may unconsciously spend more time discussing cheaper alternatives—even if those cheaper alternatives are not first-line treatments. Because providers are not conscious of their implicit thoughts, they might not realize this unless the patient has high health literacy and specifically asks about other treatment options.

One specific way that implicit bias influences clinical decisions is that physicians and other health care providers with high levels of unconscious bias often have a misperception of patient preferences. This is a common theme in Chapters 10 and 11, as disabled patients or very obese people frequently do not receive recommended preventive services based on the premise that the patient would not want them or that they would be too distressing to the patient. The way that clinicians offer or ask about a service can be influenced by their implicit biases or preferences.

For example, I once heard a gynecologist lamenting about how difficult it is to perform pelvic examinations on very large women. Her language soon turned towards discussing how these exams are not just difficult, but actually "unpleasant." Even though this is an explicit thought, her assertion that providing this service for a patient is unpleasant for *her* means that she is probably at high risk for also implicitly preferring to avoid pelvic examinations on so-called morbidly obese women. She might use language like this when a patient is due for a routine gynecological examination:

> *"We could do a PAP smear if you want, but it might be kind of difficult. Do you think you're high risk? Do you think you need it, or do you want to do it today? We could always do it later."*

Contrast this to a physician who does not have a preference for patients based on body habitus—i.e., no implicit bias for non-obese patients and no implicit bias against obese patients—and their language with the patient might be quite different:

> *"You are due for your PAP smear, and we strongly recommend it as an important part of your preventive health. Are you okay if we do that today?"*

You will probably agree that the patient of the second provider is much more likely to receive the recommended service based on the language of the physician. Pelvic examinations can be physically and emotionally uncomfortable for many patients, so a confident recommendation to receive the service might be very important for them to accept these exams. Why would a patient go through a stressful or unpleasant procedure if the provider does not seem to think it is important or does not seem to want to do it? In addition to biased words and language, implicit bias is often accompanied by body language that influences how people are perceived by others.

If a doctor appears to be repulsed or annoyed by having to provide a service, then the patient could be inclined towards declining that service. This is one way that health disparities in certain groups are perpetuated, as we will see repeatedly in this book. In addition, the "blame" will often be placed on the patient for making an unwise medical decision or rejecting a diagnostic test that was offered to them.

Implicit biases often worsen in stressful situations or when there are time constraints, such as times when the census is high on the inpatient wards of a hospital, or when a busy clinic is running an hour behind.[9] During these times, we tend to rely on ingrained assumptions about people to make quick decisions, and patients can become targets of a clinician's frustration or desire to find a shortcut. This is one example of a time when unconscious bias can affect provider feelings about, attitudes towards, and treatment of patients, resulting in lower patient satisfaction, which is one component of the "triple aim" of healthcare—that is, to (1) improve the patient experience, (2) provide high-quality care that improves the health of populations, and (3) reduce per capita cost and eliminate waste in healthcare.[10,11]

Implicit bias also interferes with an emerging recommendation to expand the triple aim into the "quadruple aim" or even the "quintuple aim." The quadruple aim includes increased satisfaction in the health care provider's experience of delivering medical care. Helping providers become aware of their implicit biases may be more satisfying once they realize that certain interactions were unconsciously distressing them and that they have the means to correct behaviors that were leading to subpar care. The quintuple aim adds the goal of also achieving health equity for populations, which is the focus of this book. Although a lot of our health equity framework focuses on systems rather than individual behavior, uncorrected implicit bias interferes with the on-the-ground application of interventions that improve the health of communities.

A classic study by Schulman et al. used a computerized survey of clinical vignettes to assess physicians' recommendations for percutaneous coronary intervention to manage a patient's chest pain.[12] When presented with patients of similar ages who have similar baseline heart disease risk, similar types of chest pain, and similar diagnostic test results, women and Black patients were less likely to receive a recommendation for cardiac catheterization. If two patients present the exact same way, and the only thing distinguishing them from each other is race or sex, then it raises a concern that implicit bias is contributing to their decision-making.

I once presented this study to a group of colleagues and was met with unexpected anger from someone with whom I had previously enjoyed a cordial relationship. This study was first published in the *New England Journal of Medicine* in 1999, and I presented it a few years after that. This was well before my health equity journey began, so I remember feeling disappointed that I had allowed myself to be fooled by what my coworker referred to as a low-quality study.

What I discovered later was that, regardless of one's thoughts about this study of cardiac catheterization recommendations, the results behind it were reproduced repeatedly in several different clinical settings. That same year, a study by Abreu in the *Journal of Consulting and Clinical Psychology* demonstrated that when health professionals were "primed" with African American stereotype-laden words, they were more likely to evaluate patients negatively.[13] Borkhoff and others presented orthopedic surgeons and family physicians with clinical vignettes of patients with unilateral knee osteoarthritis that differed only by gender, and women were less likely to be recommended for surgical repair;[14] this is supported by epidemiological data that women are three times less likely than men to receive knee arthroplasty for similar clinical presentations.[15]

When physicians are presented with patients who are essentially identical except for race and gender, they tend to make significantly different choices for and have different assumptions [think, bias!] of certain demographics of people. In a study by van Ryan and Burke, they demonstrated that, even after adjusting for income, education, personal characteristics, etc., doctors were more likely to rate Black patients as less intelligent, more likely to abuse drugs and alcohol, less likely to adhere to medical advice, more likely to lack social support, and less likely to participate in cardiac rehab.[16] Those last three assumptions support a theme that we discussed above that implicit bias can influence diagnostic and treatment decisions, and it can also create a misperception of patient preferences.

I can remember patients of mine who needed a surgical intervention, but they were declined by the surgeon for fear that the person would not be a good postoperative rehab candidate—not because of frailty or medical concerns, but just because that was the surgeon's gut feeling based on a single interaction with the patient.

I have personally had medical students and resident physicians evaluate a patient then tell me that the patient either declined a medication or diagnostic test, or that the patient did not seem interested in the recommended service. Then, when I would enter the room, the patient would immediately ask me which pharmacy they could get their prescription from, or when we were going to do their lab test. This has often been met with surprise from my junior colleagues who have sometimes defensively said, "I thought you told me that you didn't want to do that." My confused patients' responses have ranged anywhere from apologetic—for miscommunicating—to annoyed that their preferences were being misrepresented.

As I discussed at the beginning of this chapter, I am not presenting this information from a superior moral viewpoint, mocking my medical students or surgical consultants for their high levels of implicit bias. By nature, implicit bias is unconscious, so it is difficult for me to know about all the times that I assuredly make assumptions about people or prefer to be around certain people without consciously acknowledging why. In fact, there are plenty of times that I see a patient for a return visit, and I question why I made certain decisions or did not offer certain services until now. The good thing about implicit bias is that, once it is recognized and becomes explicit, most people attempt to correct the behavior.

BIAS-REDUCING STRATEGIES

One of the most effective ways to reduce implicit bias in healthcare is simply to *increase awareness* in a way that is nonjudgmental and highlights the universal nature of the problem. We all have it—we are all biased in some way—and our goal should be to find our personal blind spots while also researching the common ways that unconscious bias appears in our particular lines of work. Learning about health disparities that exist in specific medical specialties is therefore a critical task that should be done while simultaneously exploring individual bias. For example, if you are an orthopedic surgeon, then being aware that women are less likely to receive surgery for knee arthritis is an extremely important first step.

Most physicians (and most healthcare organizations) want to provide high-quality care, and you will be hard pressed to find a physician who purposefully wants women in the population to suffer from knee pain. By becoming aware of this health disparity, a surgeon is more likely to be aware of stereotypes that are thought to contribute to inequities in orthopedic care for women—such as the idea that men need surgery more because of the typical tasks that they perform and the activities that they are involved in, or that the very women who birth children are somehow less able to tolerate postoperative pain than men.

In addition to increasing awareness of implicit bias, adopting the skill of *individuating* is another important action. Individuating involves making a conscious effort to focus on specific information about an individual, which will help to override assumptions that we make about them based on their social category. One of the easiest ways to do this is to develop consistent routines and make a deliberate decision to always attempt to stick to them. Most clinicians who perform medical procedures have consistent routines that they develop during their training or shortly afterwards. On the other hand, patient interactions, counseling, and clinical decision-making are sometimes less predictable and more prone to unconscious influences.

Take, for example, the seventeen years of my career that I regularly did rounds in the newborn nursery. Early on, I developed a habit of always discussing the same issues with parents: safe sleep practices, shaken baby syndrome, avoiding smoke exposure, smoke detectors and guns in the home (or just general home safety), fevers in the first month of life, and dietary recommendations based on whether they were breast or bottle feeding.

I once came out of a room with a pair of new parents that I had also seen while serving as part of their prenatal care team. Upon exiting the hospital room, one of the resident physicians on the team remarked, "I was just telling the medical students that you say the same five or six things to every single parent, but that was the first time I didn't hear you say hardly any of them." My initial reaction was that I could not believe that I would have provided subpar counseling and anticipatory guidance to this family that I had a positive relationship with, but fortunately the encounter had just happened moments earlier.

As a result, I was able to recall the details easily and realized that the resident was correct; I provided a very thorough examination and discussed the case in detail with the team, but my counseling was not typical. The mother was on her cell phone and would not get off. When I told her that we could come back, she asked me to go on and talk while she clearly continued to listen to the person on the other end of the phone call. I recalled how these parents previously seemed to blow off my advice about not smoking around their children and trying to quit before this child was born. My unconscious thoughts became conscious (i.e., "explicit") at that moment, as I realized that I cut out some of my counseling for these parents because I did not think they cared.

Now, you may be thinking that it is a waste of time to keep talking to someone who is not listening, and that I was not in the wrong for giving up after a genuine attempt to have the mother's undivided attention. This is not, however, the great realization that I came to on that day; my epiphany was not related to the way I sometimes respond to people preoccupied with their cell phones. *I realized that I had a strong implicit bias against people who smoke cigarettes.* The first thought that came to my mind after my resident's critique was, *Those parents never really seemed to care about their health, so why should I put in more effort than they do?*

Fortunately, I did not say those thoughts out loud to my team of students and residents, and I was disturbed by the ideas that had entered my mind and caused me to rush out of the room prematurely. I knew that I always had a high level of disdain for tobacco companies, as cigarettes have been the leading cause of preventable death over my lifetime.[17] I was concerned that my attitudes had spread over to the consumers of these companies' products as well.

Over the next few weeks, I began to critique my encounters with tobacco smokers in my outpatient practice and on the inpatient service during the periods that I served as the supervising physician. Another surprising scenario arose when one of my patients who was a smoker was seen by a colleague of mine, and they were giving me an update on the patient. They mentioned counseling her extensively about her smoking, and they laughed because the patient said that I did not really ever talk to her about smoking. My coworker told me that their response to the patient was, "Dr. Reddick hates smoking more than anyone I know. There's no way he hasn't talked to you about smoking." Unfortunately, the patient was probably right.

I began to realize how my mind would often doubt that smokers would make healthy lifestyle choices based merely on their tobacco abuse, and I also had a high level of doubt about my own abilities to help them become abstinent from cigarettes. When I saw patients with lung cancer or end-stage emphysema who continued to smoke, my lack of confidence would sometimes turn into an abundance of frustration. Using our definition of implicit bias above, I definitely fit the bill of a biased individual with a strong preference for patients who did not smoke cigarettes and a preference to not have the exasperation felt when caring for patients who could not quit smoking.

The silver lining of these anecdotes is that they were the beginning of a new approach to the clinical care that I provide. While I had always attempted to provide the same high-quality care to all patients, I was easily thrown off by implicit biases against certain groups—smokers in this most recent example. I learned the skill of *individuating*, and I made a more conscious effort to not lump each patient from a group together, but rather to give each individual the same opportunities and options that everyone else has. I had previously developed a counseling routine in the newborn nursery for *most* parents, but I would make assumptions about which ones were ready to receive it.

When my unconscious attitudes and beliefs became conscious, I began to do a better job of presenting the same information to everyone and allowing them to make decisions without passing judgment on my part. I tapped into some of the skills that we learned in our medical training, such as motivational interviewing and the transtheoretical model of health behavior change.[18] I also began to review the evidence-based approaches to smoking cessation more aggressively, and I began to make a conscious effort to try and remember to offer these to every patient of mine who smokes. I also began to take stock whenever I was knocked off my usual course of action or counseling, and I would look for any unconscious thoughts that might have caused this change on my part.

The bias-reducing strategy of *perspective-taking* becomes even more important in Chapter 3 as we explore explicit biases, but it is also critical in that initial moment when implicit biases become explicit or conscious. When discussing intersectionality in the Preface and Chapter 1, I mentioned that each person responds differently to similar life events. Likewise, there are a combination of physical, environmental, and social forces that determine which people respond to adversity or challenges in a manner that we deem socially desirable. Use of perspective-taking to be more empathetic and less judgmental has even been recommended by national experts such as Dr. Quinn Capers in non-clinical settings such as medical school admissions.[19]

Whenever we have difficulty removing negative thoughts and reactions towards someone based on their personal decisions or life circumstances, we should consider what life events or societal influences may have contributed to that person's situation and choices. We should also delve into our own psyche to see what life experiences have created biases within ourselves. Let us look at the example of my own past bias against cigarette smokers. Where did this come from, and how did I use it to become more empathetic towards smokers?

My father grew up in rural North Carolina working on tobacco farms, and he began smoking cigarettes as an adolescent. Those were the days when the dangers of smoking were not as obvious to the public, and he was addicted to nicotine before he learned about the harms of tobacco. As a young child, my siblings and I would walk around the house obnoxiously praying out loud, "God, please help Dad quit smoking before he dies." Eventually he was able to quit after just going "cold turkey" one day, and I was convinced from childhood that any human could choose to tap into that same willpower if they really wanted to stop smoking. Furthermore, I was less sympathetic towards people who began smoking in recent years, when the surgeon general's warnings and widespread knowledge of the dangers of cigarettes are everywhere. I am pretty sure that this contributed to why I was so hard on other people in the past who could not quit smoking. In my mind, they just did not try hard enough or did not care enough about their health.

What I did not consider until recent years was whether my father would have quit smoking if he had been a single man without bratty children who pestered him on a daily basis about his cigarettes. Or whether it would have been as easy for him to quit if he had several other health behaviors that he was trying to change simultaneously. Or whether he would have had as much success at getting rid of cigarettes if he was not an attorney with good health literacy and access to a medical provider who was also counseling him to quit.

Social support is an important component of a plan to change multiple risk behaviors,[20] and the COVID-19 pandemic has increased social isolation for a lot of my patients. Perspective-taking requires exploring who people are, and how they ended up where they are, in a non-condemnatory way. Instead of trying to scare people into quitting smoking or telling them about the harms of smoking, understanding what they enjoy about smoking and why they began smoking is probably a better first step. We will explore the concept of harm reduction in Chapter 13 with a focus on improving the health of people who use drugs using a judgment-free and evidence-based approach; this framework will be useful for counseling patients about legal and illegal drug use.

You can see how my previous smorgasbord of stereotyping and unconscious bias led to the potential harms that we discussed earlier: assumptions about patient preference, incorrectly interpreting their thoughts and motivations, worsening of these feelings during times of stress, and interference with the delivery of high-quality care. What I failed to do in the past was what sounds like a cliché…trying to walk a mile in their shoes.

KNOWLEDGE, ATTITUDES, AND SKILLS

Knowledge

- We *all* have implicit biases, which are preferences for or against particular groups of people. These biases are unconscious, so the person holding them is unaware of these thoughts until they are brought to light by another person or by introspection.

- Every one of our biases, even ones based on preferences for groups or based on "positive" stereotypes, have the potential to harm someone either in the affected group or in the excluded group.

- Unconscious bias causes physicians and other health care providers to make potentially false assumptions about patient preferences, and these assumptions may influence the diagnostic and treatment options that are offered to patients.

- Clinicians who have high levels of bias have lower rates of patient satisfaction, and their negative behavior tends to increase during times of high stress or when there are significant time limitations.

Attitudes

- Although healthcare is generally viewed as an altruistic career, systematic reviews have demonstrated that health care professionals have the same levels of implicit bias as the general population.[21] We are not special!

- We should embrace diversity and enjoy spending time with people who are different than us, especially those who are from groups that we have not had much interaction with. Being around people outside of our usual circle can counter conscious and unconscious stereotypes that we may be harboring.

- Being aware of cultural differences and trends in certain populations is normal, but we should remember that every person from those groups does not fit these generalizations and images that we have in our minds.

Skills

- Increase awareness of health disparities that exist within your medical specialty, as most of us will look to counter any inequities that we contribute to.

- Make a conscious effort to focus on specific information about the patient in front of you. Treat each person like an individual; this means offering everyone the same high-quality care and counseling, but also being flexible, understanding, and nonjudgmental when someone makes a choice that you do not understand.

- Perform perpetual self-assessment and reflection to look for implicit biases, especially whenever you have a negative or distressing encounter with another person.

- Implement perspective-taking and consciously attempt to envision the other person's viewpoint whenever you are at an impasse. If their behavior is confusing to you, then get to know them and explore how they arrived at their current place in life.

HOW TO TEACH ABOUT IMPLICIT BIAS

Here is one of my favorite ways to teach about implicit bias, especially for people who are skeptical of the concept. Put the following photograph (Image 1), or one like it, into a PowerPoint or other visual presentation:

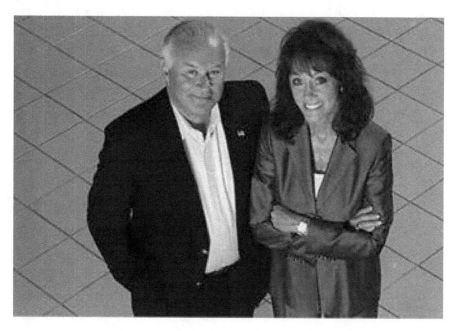

First, inform the audience that you are going to do an exercise to demonstrate both implicit and explicit biases that they may be harboring. Tell them that this is a picture of a billionaire who paid $0 in taxes over at least a three-year period. Next, ask the audience to pretend that this billionaire came to you asking you to do a favor for their son. If you are a faculty member at a medical school or residency program, pretend that they asked you to help their son with mediocre grades to get in. If you work at an outpatient office, pretend that they asked you to get their son some samples for asthma inhalers because their insurance copay recently increased to $60. Finally, ask the audience if they have any explicit biases against this billionaire, or if you think there is any chance that they have unconscious biases against someone like this.

I have done this activity at least two dozen times, and I have received several disparaging remarks about the gentleman in the photograph. I have heard him referred to as smug, had people criticize his tan, and the majority of my audiences have said that they would refuse to help him. The funny thing about this photograph is that…*the man is not the billionaire!* This is an actual photograph of Diane Kendricks, a billionaire from Wisconsin, along with her husband; she is the one who came under fire a few years ago when it was announced that she did not pay any state income tax for three years.[22]

Most people that I encounter do not recognize her just from a snapshot, if they have ever heard of her at all, so this works well. If you know of any other women billionaires that the average person would not recognize, then a picture of them standing next to a man should suffice. Pictures of Oprah Winfrey next to her longtime partner (Stedman Graham) would probably not work.

The point of this exercise is not to have a discussion about taxes or wealth inequality, and you should feel comfortable to steer the conversation away from that if it takes such a turn. The point is that people hear "billionaire" and assume it is the man. Notice that, in the picture above, the husband and wife appear to be the same height, they are both smiling, and they are equally spaced. I also used gender-neutral pronouns the entire time in describing the scenario, but people always assume I am talking about the man. We hear about someone rich and think about a man, similar to how people often hear the name of a doctor and think of a man. This implicit bias can affect what kind of people we imagine in certain careers, be it as a physician, as a nurse, or as a hospital executive.

Out of the more than twenty times that I have staged this activity, I only remember maybe two times that someone asked, "Which one is the billionaire?" If this happens, you can still accomplish the goal of the exercise by asking the audience to be honest and raise their hands if they assumed that the man was the billionaire. The one or two times this happened, almost everyone in the room raised their hands and admitted that they unconsciously assumed that it was the man.

The most memorable version of this training involved a participant who proclaimed at the onset that he does not have any biases and thought that it was sad that we needed this type of education. During this "billionaire" portion of the talk, he reminded the group that he has no biases and told me that he would not hold it against the man's son if his father came off as a bit greedy to some. I had the immense joy of telling him, "But the man isn't the billionaire," followed by the explanation that he had just demonstrated an implicit bias.

The stunned look on his face was priceless and the audience erupted in laughter. He briefly argued that I must have used masculine pronouns at some point, but the audience corroborated my assertion that I had not. Remember, however, that the point of these activities is not to embarrass anyone. In short manner, I followed up with an explanation that we all do this, and I told him about one of my recent encounters with a patient when I demonstrated similar assumptions subconsciously. My patient told me that they were referred to a cardiologist during a recent hospitalization, and I asked what *he* recommended. My patient responded, "Doc, the heart doctor was a 'she.'"

CHAPTER 3

EXPLICIT BIAS AND RACISM

DR. BONZO'S BUNGLE OF THE MONTH:
Prejudiced Against Drug Reps?

Between the time consumed by my career, my children, and other family responsibilities, my wife and I have tried to consciously carve out time to spend with each other sans children. During one of our "date nights," we attended a comedy show hosted by a family friend who I have known since childhood. We had the opportunity to hang out backstage with my buddy, and I began chatting with a guy who was friends with another one of the performers. The conversation started out with comedy as the main subject, but it quickly morphed into sports and a number of other shared interests. I introduced him to my wife, who was standing nearby, and he mentioned that we should get together for a double dinner date soon. We were both avid runners and shared similar workout routines, so we also discussed doing some training together in the near future.

He asked me about my career, and he seemed interested in what my job as a physician was like; he specifically asked me if I ever had to deal with "drug reps." Since he asked if I had to "deal with them" I assumed he had a negative view of these reps, so I told him that I was thrilled when our clinic stopped hosting representatives of the pharmaceutical industry. I unleashed about how annoying they are and told him that "I can't stand them." We proceeded to talk about his occupation, and of course when I asked what his wife does, he told me, "She's a drug rep." Oops! Needless to say, the conversation ended awkwardly, and my wife and I never hung out with that couple.

I believe that most people will be sympathetic towards my bungle from Chapter 2, because it came from a place of wanting to help others. After reading this one, you might be thinking, "Wow, this Dr.

Bonzo guy is a jerk." Well, let us look at the source of my explicit bias against industry reps and see how this developed into me inadvertently insulting a stranger's wife. Over the years, I had become increasingly convinced by medical literature that demonstrated how pharmaceutical companies strive to manipulate physicians into prescribing their medications while simultaneously convincing the lay public that they need to ask their doctors to prescribe these medications.[1] After learning how this results in increased prescribing and increased costs without any improvement in health outcomes, I ultimately agreed with the American Medical Association (AMA) who called for a ban of direct-to-consumer advertising for prescription drugs—a practice that is banned in most countries around the world.[2,3]

One of the last meaningful interactions that I had with a pharmaceutical sales rep prior to our clinic's shift away from hosting them involved a gentleman who was marketing a long-acting insulin brand. He repeatedly showed up to our clinic to provide lunch for our residents, medical students, and clinic staff, and he would hang out in the back of our conference room during the moments before our didactic sessions began. I almost always pack my own lunch and did not eat his meals, so I did not feel obligated to talk to him. He was not aggressive in his approach, and he was so polite to me that it became increasingly difficult to give him the cold shoulder; so, I at least began to be cordial with him.

One day, this drug rep was discussing his long-acting insulin with a group of medical students, explaining how his insulin lasts a full 24 hours, not 23.9 hours like their leading competitor (of course I am being facetious here, but you get the point). He discussed with our students that some patients are even able to obtain control of their diabetes just by using this once-a-day, long-acting insulin without the need for three additional doses of mealtime insulin. This part of the conversation sparked a bit of interest in me because I had recently prescribed this brand of insulin in that exact manner for a patient with a serious mental health disorder and a mild fear of needles.

The patient was a newly diagnosed diabetic, and they were distressed that they would have to administer four injections per day.

I ultimately decided to try just a single dose of long-acting insulin along with the oral medication metformin, a process that the drug rep had described. I told my patient that they would really have to work on their diet and begin an exercise routine if they wanted to avoid the three additional mealtime insulin injections. The psychiatric team set the patient up with some community resources for supervised exercise, and the patient had excellent results.

By the time of this patient's three-month follow-up, their diabetes was under excellent control, and soon afterwards I ran into our drug rep during one of his marketing visits. He remembered the discussion about my patient and asked how things were going; he was thrilled to hear about the success story and quickly shared it with anyone who was within earshot. My patient embraced this lifestyle change and became enthralled by their new exercise routine; their psychiatrist even mentioned that the patient's behavioral health had significantly improved with this improvement in their metabolic state. When I was able to wean the patient off their long-acting insulin a few months later, their joy and elation would have made you think that they had just won the championship!

You might see where things are going, but fast forward to the next time that I ran into the drug rep. He again wanted to know how my patient was doing. I was proud to tell him that they no longer needed the long-acting insulin, as my patient had gone from a double-digit hemoglobin A1c value to an A1c below 6 percent after losing weight and exercising regularly; he remained well-controlled at all follow-ups after switching to a regimen of just an oral medication. My drug rep was extremely disappointed and began lecturing me that, "all diabetics need a little basal insulin. You should put him on *just a little touch of insulin* so that he doesn't go backwards."

Although I always kind of knew, it became crystal clear at that exact moment that this drug rep's only goal was to get me to prescribe his insulin, and he would even stoop to giving me inaccurate medical advice to make this happen—advice that is potentially harmful given the risk of hypoglycemia, or low blood sugar, in this situation that he recommended.

He could sense how annoyed I had become in that moment, so he began telling me that he could put me in touch with the chief of endocrinology at Ivy League University—not the real name of the university that he quoted, sorry for being facetious again—who would tell me that leaving on this patient's insulin and backing off their oral medication was a smart plan. I declined, ended the conversation, and never spoke to him again. This chapter's bungle at the comedy show happened shortly after this final drug rep interaction.

The point of this detailed story was not to justify my rude behavior to the gentleman (and his wife) at the comedy show or to rationalize my explicit bias against pharmaceutical reps. This anecdote shows how a bias can insidiously build until an interaction that was simply annoying and disappointing could cause me to make an insulting remark in public shortly afterwards without considering that someone nearby could be hurt by my comments. Remarkably, I cannot recall ever having a patient who was an industry rep but, shortly after pondering this interaction, I wondered how my past biases against them would have affected the care that I provided if I had patients who represented the prescription drug industry.

I can recall a clinical encounter many years ago when I was a medical student and a patient's father let it be known that he was a drug rep. He began asking for specific brands of medication for his child, which clearly annoyed my attending physician. My teaching physician refused to prescribe one of the brand-named medications that the father asked for, saying that another brand was equally as good—and this was true, both treatments were first-line—and that allowing patients to dictate clinician prescribing practices is not a good thing. I can imagine that the old Dr. Bonzo would have reacted the same way.

Think about how much worse my behavior and words might have been at the comedy show if I had been physically harmed by a drug rep, or if drug reps had stolen things from me in the past. These are the same justifications that people use to defend their dislike of people based on skin color or sexual orientation. When I saw this parallel between how I reacted to a profession and how people react to other groups of people, I made a conscious effort to try and never disparage a group of people, no matter how inconsequential my words may seem at the time. (The one group that I am still struggling with in this regard are the people who run tobacco companies, but I am working on it.)

The people who market pharmaceutical products are not a group that is known to collectively experience health inequities but, at the individual level, bias against any person for any reason will likely interfere with the patient-doctor relationship and can lead to lower quality care. The target groups described in this book are prone to widespread explicit biases against them, which can have even more harmful effects than the implicit biases described in the previous chapter.

REVIEW OF DEFINITIONS AND NEW TERMINOLOGY

In Chapter 2, we defined *implicit bias* as an unconscious preference for or against a particular group of people, while *explicit biases* are deliberately formed predilections.[4,5] These biases either form based on our past experiences with the groups that we prefer to be around or prefer to avoid, or they are based on a lack of experience with these groups. Biases are usually accompanied by unverified assumptions about people—called *stereotypes*—that are based on generalizations that are sometimes present in society but are often exaggerated or misrepresented in media representations of these groupings. When our biases become antagonistic or hostile and linked to negative stereotypes, we refer to them as *prejudices*.[6]

A person can be prejudiced against any of the target groups that we discuss in this book, and there are general terms that most people use to identify these discriminatory thoughts and behaviors. Hostile and negative explicit biases against people based on race or ethnicity is often defined as racism, prejudice against women is often referred to as sexism, discrimination against disabled people is often called ableism, and bigotry against sexual and gender minorities is often termed homophobia or transphobia. This chapter explores racism in detail, and the other themes also each have dedicated chapters later in this book.

Racism is most commonly defined as a belief that a certain racial or ethnic group is inherently inferior to another group, whereas others are inherently superior (either biologically or culturally); the term racism also typically encompasses hatred towards these racial or ethnic groups. Dr. Camara Jones is often credited with introducing a new definition of racism into the lexicon of medicine and public health. *Systemic racism*—also known as *structural racism*—is a system of structuring opportunity and assigning value based on the social interpretation of how one looks.[7] Whereas *individual racism* requires a person to consciously dislike a race of people or believe that they are superior to this racial group, *systemic racism* does not require a conscious or intentional foundation—although many systems of racism may have been initially created purposefully.

Systemic racism simply means that certain racial and ethnic groups have more opportunities or are deemed more valuable by the system; therefore, other groups have fewer opportunities and are considered less valuable systemically. Chapter 1 describes how intent does not matter in these situations, as patients are still harmed by systemic racism in healthcare, and it also describes that focusing too much on individual behavior distracts from the need to fix *systems*.

In addition to distracting from systemic issues, another reason that I typically avoid conversations about individual racism is that *no one will ever admit that they are a racist!* Three police officers in Wilmington, North Carolina—a city where I lived for four years—were fired in 2020 after unknowingly being recorded at work while expressing a desire to commit genocide against Black people. These details plus more are depicted in an article by Tim Elfrink of *The Washington Post*, which also describes how one of the officers, Kevin Piner, discussed plans to buy high-powered weaponry and "slaughter" Black people.[8] They predicted that a civil war would follow the protests for racial equality that occurred after the death of George Floyd and others.

The officer said, "I'm ready…We are just going to go out and start slaughtering them f--k-ng n-gg-rs." He also said that he wanted to "wipe [Black people] off the f--k-ng map" with the hopes that his actions would "put 'em back about four or five generations." This former cop somehow managed to completely embody individual and systemic racism in one sentence. He expressed the excitement and anticipation of a child waiting for Christmas gifts as he said, "God, I can't wait." All three of these police officers were hired in either 1997 or 1998, so they each had more than twenty years on the job which must have included countless encounters with Black people.

So, what was the reaction of these three police officers when they were confronted with audiovisual copies of these recordings?

1. They admitted it was their voices on the recording.
2. They did not deny any of the content or say that the words were misinterpreted.
3. *They denied that they were racists!*

This exemplifies why accusing people of individual racism is an exercise in futility, and I do not know how to fix a behavior that people will always deny even exists. To date, I have never heard a person admit that they are racist.

EXPLICIT BIAS AND SYSTEMIC RACISM IN HEALTHCARE

A study of fourth-year medical students by Harrison et al. found that they had significant explicit biases against obese people, patients of low socioeconomic status, and patients who smoke.[9] (The previous chapter described how I was also once guilty of this.) They also had low levels of explicit biases against some patients based on race and ethnicity. Whereas people will rarely admit to embracing racist ideals, stereotypes of racial and ethnic groups are not considered as socially unacceptable by some segments of the population. For example, in the IOM's *Unequal Treatment* report, they described surveys among White Americans whereby anywhere from 50–75 percent believe that Black people are less intelligent, more prone to violence, and prefer to live off welfare.[5] While the majority of this chapter focuses on adjusting systems to combat bias, this chapter does discuss how to challenge and reduce individual explicit biases and also how to counter the stereotypes that accompany these biases.

There are endless studies going back more than two decades that demonstrate instances of systemic racism in healthcare. In studies of acute low back pain, Black patients were perceived by health care providers to have less severe pain, and they received less radiographs and advanced imaging studies despite presenting with worse functional status.[10] These disparities persist even after controlling for income, education, pain score (baseline severity of the patient's low back pain), and insurance status. White patients are more likely than Black patients to be treated with opioids for chronic pain, even when they present with similar injuries or report similar pain scores.[11] While it can be argued that radiographic studies and opioid analgesia are overused in this country, the concern is that one segment of the population is not offered the same diagnostic and treatment options as another—something that, as we learned in Chapter 2, happens when clinicians have high levels of implicit bias.

The pediatric medical literature also describes unequal treatment for acutely painful medical conditions based on the patients' race. In a retrospective cohort study of more than 20,000 patients with long bone fractures, non-Latino White children were more likely to receive opioid analgesia for similar injuries.[12] Black children were 30 percent less likely to receive opioids, while Hispanic children were 28 percent less likely. In the National Hospital Ambulatory Medical Care Survey, conducted from 2003 to 2010, a cross-sectional study of more than 900,000 cases of acute appendicitis also showed unequal administration of narcotic pain medication.[13] While the overall rate of analgesia in this study was the same between races, Black children and adolescents with severe pain were less likely to receive opioids than White children. Think of a Black child receiving ibuprofen for acute appendicitis, while a White child reporting the same pain level receives morphine.

The IOM report revealed some of the stereotypes and explicit beliefs that frequently exist with regard to racial and ethnic minorities.

African American and Hispanic people are often labeled as being more likely to abuse drugs despite the fact that their drug use is typically the same or lower than the rates for the general population.[14,15] This could translate into an unsubstantiated fear of prescribing opioid pain medications to Black and Latino patients. I doubt that emergency room physicians and nurses go to work each day with the goal of withholding pain medication from racial and ethnic minorities, but these examples likely demonstrate how implicit and explicit biases result in substandard care. They also highlight why systemic changes are needed to overcome individual behaviors and practices.

One of the most disturbing instances of systemic racism in healthcare is related to the maternal mortality rate of Black women in the United States, which has ranged between three to four times higher than the rate for White women in recent years. This country is one of the few in the world that has seen an increase in maternal mortality over the past fifteen years, and it has consistently had the worst rate of industrially developed countries. Despite this dreary backdrop, the maternal mortality rate of African American women still stands out, as they are significantly more likely to die during pregnancy or within the year after they give birth compared to their American counterparts of other races.

The maternal mortality rate in my home state of Georgia has been so dismal over the past decade that it was flagged by Amnesty International, and the Yale Global Health Justice Partnership (GHJP) published a special report on how to address this health inequity.[16] The Yale GHJP is a joint endeavor between Yale School of Public Health and Yale Law School, and one of their goals was to develop policies and programs to promote health justice. In the case of Georgia, they described four *systemic* issues that contribute to the bleak maternal mortality rate:

1. Barriers to accessing high-quality prenatal care in a timely manner

2. Inadequate and inconsistent insurance coverage

3. Lack of funding for maternal health

4. A Maternal Mortality Review Committee (MMRC) that provides only the bare minimum in tracking, investigating, and intervening upon maternal deaths.

Going back to our definition of systemic racism, the result is a racist system that disadvantages people of a certain racial or ethnic group. It does not matter whether individual people are harboring racist values while these statewide policies are implemented.

In the case of Georgia's MMRC, meeting the national minimum standard of competency did not adequately address or reverse the problem. The Yale GHJP described how the membership of the Committee was not made public which resulted in a lack of transparency or accountability. They only released one report over several years, and they failed to focus on the role of social determinants of health in driving health inequities. (Chapter 9 will highlight why this was a critical oversight.) Their reporting system had limited funding and lacked research and forensic capacity, which has a direct impact on the ability to assess the root causes when maternal deaths do occur. Combating systemic racism often requires going above the existing minimum standards, which makes perfect sense when you consider that those standards were created by the racist system.

Now, contrast the situation in Georgia with the maternal mortality trend in the state of California.[17] Their state's Department of Public Health (DPH) began a rigorous investigation in 2004 to explore the rise in maternal deaths. Two years later, they formed their version of a MMRC, the California Maternal Quality Care Collaborative (CMQCC) at Stanford University School of Medicine, not only to report the causes of these deaths but also to identify solutions.[18] They linked hospital discharge and birth certificate data so that they were able to obtain data for approximately 95 percent of all births in California.[19]

Their goal was to reduce the incidence of all types of maternal deaths, but the CMQCC particularly focused on ways to reduce deaths from some of the major contributors: obstetric hemorrhage, high cesarean section rates, venous thromboembolism (VTE), cardiovascular disease, maternal suicide, and hypertensive disorders of pregnancy such as preeclampsia. One of the most important interventions was the development of toolkits that were disseminated to hospitals around the state with guidance on how to prevent these drivers of maternal mortality—or to at least intervene quickly when they appear.

The result was that California's maternal mortality decreased by 55 percent over the eight-year period between 2006 and 2013— from 16.9 deaths per 100,000 births to 7.3 deaths per 100,000 births (Image 2). This means that California went from a rate that was 3.6 [per 100,000] *above* the national average to a rate that was 14.7 [per 100,000] *below* the national average, even as rates around the country continued to increase. In addition to decreased mortality, California has experienced a decrease in indicators of morbidity, including a

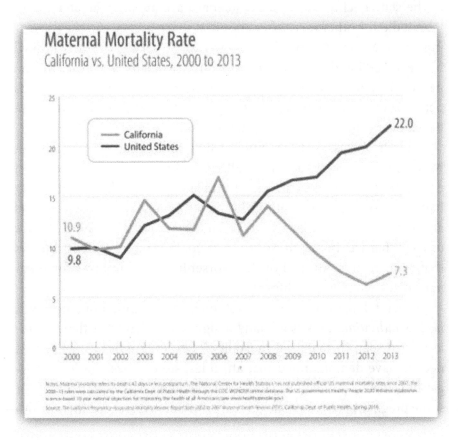

more than 20 percent decline in the cesarean section rate after implementation of a six-month pilot in 2014. California has strived to create the transparency recommended by the Yale GHJP; case reports on pregnancy-related deaths between 2008 and 2016 are available to the public on the CMQCC website, as are the names and pictures of all committee members.

Now, you may be wondering what this obstetric success story in California has to do with racial health inequities or systemic racism. As mentioned earlier, the maternal mortality rate for Black women in the United States has tripled and even quadrupled the rate for White women at times, so an overall decrease in mortality does not necessarily mean that racial inequities are improving. In the case of California, however, this is exactly what it meant.

As Image 3 illustrates, the maternal death rates for Black women in the state declined at a much steeper pace and to a greater extent than it did for other races after an initial sharp increase in the preceding years. Maternal mortality for African American women peaked between 2005 and 2007, when it astonishingly surpassed fifty maternal deaths per 100,000 live births despite rates well below 15 deaths per 100,000 for all other racial groups. By 2013, the rate of Black maternal deaths had decreased by nearly half.

This is an excellent example of how addressing systemic issues resulted in a decrease in racial health inequities. When thinking about eradicating systemic racism in healthcare, you might have initially had an image of finding all of the secretly racist doctors and nurses and firing them, similar to the Wilmington, North Carolina, police officers that we discussed earlier. Instead, there were system changes that resulted in a reversal of this worsening mortality rate for pregnant Black women in California.

What I have purposefully not mentioned until now, however, is that *individual* bias is actually a significant driver of the systemic racism seen in maternal mortality.[20] Several studies over the past decade have demonstrated that attitudes, stereotypes, and biases regarding Black, Indigenous, and Latina women worsen outcomes for some pregnant patients as health care providers disregard their health

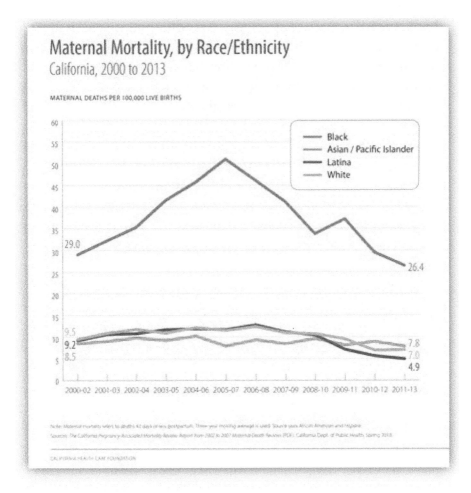

Maternal Mortality, by Race/Ethnicity
California, 2000 to 2013

MATERNAL DEATHS PER 100,000 LIVE BIRTHS

concerns or minimize their presenting symptoms.[21,22] This creates an environment that women would rather avoid even when they have medical complications or when they are in need of postpartum care.

As discussed in Chapter 2, biases and undesirable behavior worsen during periods of high stress or when there are significant time constraints. During the seventeen years that I delivered babies, I can think of several instances when I had to argue with labor and delivery nurses to begin magnesium sulfate therapy for patients with severe preeclampsia. Intravenous magnesium sulfate is the main intervention that we currently have to decrease morbidity and mortality related to preeclampsia when it presents with severe features; however, it is labor intensive to manage and does come with some notable risks and side effects. When patients seem "close to delivery" or when they "just barely meet the criteria" for preeclampsia with severe features, nurses have asked me if we could see how things go without the magnesium.

If my memory serves me correctly, every one of these instances happened when our labor and delivery units were extremely busy, never when the census was low or when things were calm. Despite this probable underlying reason for these requests, I doubt that they would ask this if these patients had been daughters of the hospital CEO. This delivery of inferior care tends to happen for people who are not as valued by society, and it demonstrates why systemic changes, protocols, and oversight are necessary to improve health outcomes for marginalized groups.

The link between bias, racism, and inferior health outcomes has been demonstrated for innumerable other medical conditions. Dr. David Williams, from the Harvard T.H. Chan School of Public Health, has published extensively on how individual-level discrimination and systemic racism are linked to worsening physical and mental health outcomes.[23] These stressors can even potentially contribute to deleterious heritable and non-heritable epigenetic changes to the genomic makeup of patients. (If you have difficulty accessing some of his journal articles, his TEDMED Talk from 2016 is available online and does an excellent job of summarizing some of these themes.)[24]

Because of the impact that individual bias has on our patients, we should continue to hold implicit bias trainings, and I will continue to discuss explicit bias as I have in this chapter; but this is only the proverbial tip of the iceberg in addressing the looming systemic bias underneath the surface. By focusing too much on individual biases, we run the risk of blaming the problem on "a few bad apples" and not employing the resources and intensity required to reduce systemic inequities. Whenever I provide implicit bias training for healthcare organizations or for my learners, I make it known that it is akin to the kindergarten of health equity education. Once we learn how to comprehensively address and overcome the factors that create a biased system, then they will be ready for graduation.

COMBATING SYSTEMIC RACISM AND MORE
BIAS-REDUCING STRATEGIES

The CMQCC in California utilized several proven techniques to combat systemic racism in healthcare and public health. Dr. Camara Jones, whose definition of systemic racism we used previously in this chapter, recommends *measuring institutional racism* as an important primary step.[7] As described above, they spent *two years* doing this in California. This should not be used as an excuse to procrastinate or drag out the process, but this analysis should be thorough and not just a cursory glance at the issues. Some of Dr. Jones' suggestions on how to accomplish this include scanning for evidence of racial disparities, identifying mechanisms or root causes of these disparities, and investigating policies that allow segregation of resources and risks. This same framework can be used for health inequities that exist beyond race and ethnicity, but the disparities that affect racial and ethnic minorities are unique based on the lack of a clear definition and understanding of race in our society.

The practice of medicine has operated as if our definitions of race have a biological construct as opposed to a social one. This concept will be explored in great detail in the next chapter, but I will briefly discuss the ramifications of our misunderstanding of the concept of race.

Dr. Nancy Krieger and colleagues described how, back in the mid- to late-1800s, Dr. James McCune Smith—the first university-trained Black physician in the United States—argued against the widespread belief that the poor health status among Black people reflected an innate genetic inferiority.[25] For example, he was able to demonstrate that the higher rates of rickets seen in the Black population was a result of poverty and poor nutrition; poor White people and poor Black people had similar rates of rickets, and rich White people had much lower rates of rickets than poor White people.

If we believe that the health disparities that exist in Black populations are the results of physiological differences between races, then it is easier to deny that racist systems are to blame. Using Dr. McCune

Smith's example, it would have been easier to (erroneously) say that Black people are genetically different and simply need more vitamin D supplementation, as opposed to exploring the systemic injustices that resulted in unequal access to nutrient-rich foods.

This fallacy of biological differences between races still exists today, and it is a possible contributor to the inequities in pain control for Black and Hispanic people described earlier in this chapter. In a study of 222 medical students at the University of Virginia School of Medicine, greater than 45 percent of those surveyed believed several race-based myths, including the idea that Black people have thicker skin and less sensitive nerve endings than other people.[26] This leads to another key step in eradicating systemic racism: *establishing a consensus on how we define and understand race.*

In my experience, it has been more of a challenge to introduce these health equity concepts once a clinician has already been practicing a certain way for a long period of time. Even third-year medical students tend to argue back that their views of race formed during the first two years of their training could not possibly be problematic. I have found that *promoting health equity and discussing systemic bias from the onset of medical education* is crucial in achieving future success as our learners will eventually become clinicians and leaders of healthcare organizations.

In an essay published in the *Journal of the American Medical Association (JAMA)* in 2015, former Brown University medical student Katherine Brooks—who I assume is Dr. Brooks by now—discussed the "silent curriculum" in medical schools.[27] Her medical educators frequently discussed racial differences in health outcomes, but they did not discuss why disparities exist or the role that racism plays in racial and ethnic inequities. She even described a "palpable discomfort" whenever a student did ask about racism.

The social determinants of health and the social construct of race are more complex to discuss than theoretical genetic or physiologic causes of health disparities, and many instructors and professors have told me that they do not have the training to discuss these complicated topics.

In addition to changing the way we review the content of medical education or the underlying theories behind how we view race, organizational structure is also a vital part of any institutional plan to eradicate systemic racism and other structural biases. Dr. David Acosta, chief diversity and inclusion officer of the AAMC, describes five principles for health equity in academic medicine:[28]

1. Proactive education about the history of exclusion of certain groups in workplace settings

2. Rejection of the habit of blaming inequities on the disadvantaged groups' social, cultural, or educational backgrounds

3. Intentionality in deconstructing the structures and systems that have sustained existing inequities

4. System-based thinking that shifts paradigms, invests in student success, and holds faculty accountable for institutional effectiveness

5. Courage to begin these discussions, truly invest in addressing health inequities, and end exclusionary practices.

The result should be the full integration and empowerment of people from all backgrounds, which will lead to increased diversity and a culture of inclusivity for the future healthcare workforce.

The AAMC Institutional Diversity Paradigm (Image 4)[29] can be applied not only to academic medical centers, but also to other healthcare organizations. The overarching theme is to develop a strategic plan that aligns the diversity mission with the institutional mission. The *goals* should be to serve diverse populations of the institution's catchment area, to expand the health care research agenda, and to prepare effective and culturally competent physicians who will care for the underserved.

Using this paradigm, the organizational *objectives* will be to obtain a critical mass of underrepresented and historically marginalized groups, to create and support structural or compositional diversity, and to enhance learning and professional development. The *strategies* that can be employed to meet these goals and objectives include outreach and pipeline programs, clinical and research initiatives, financial support (including scholarships for academic centers), holistic admissions and hiring processes, and curriculum changes that promote health equity—for non-academic medical centers; these curricular changes may be in the form of continuing medical education (CME).

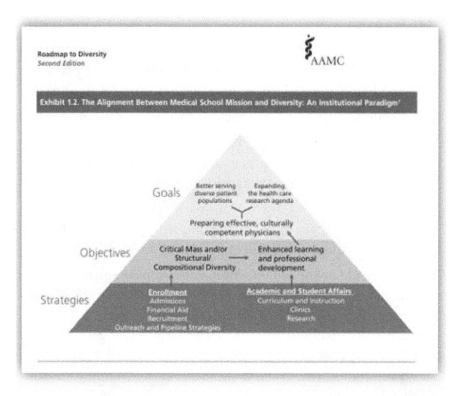

Although the lion's share of work in achieving health equity will be in addressing systemic problems, behavior that attempts to obstruct these strategies must also be addressed. This brings us to the final method of combating systemic racism and bias in healthcare: *while addressing the system, still hold individuals accountable.* Past president of the American Academy of Pediatrics (AAP), Dr. Sally Goza, did an excellent job of summarizing this when she said, "We must dismantle racism at every level, from individual to institutional to systemic."[30]

The AAP has been clear on their definition of racism—utilizing the same definition from Dr. Camara Jones that we have used here—and on their view of race as a social construct rather than a biological one; in their words, "the problem is racism, not race." They describe success with cultural diversity trainings, and they also mention the importance of educational access and attainment and the effect that this social determinant (access to high-quality education) has on health outcomes. The AAP strategies for system changes, similar to the AAMC Institutional Diversity Paradigm, include optimizing clinical practice, optimizing workforce development and professional education, optimizing research, and optimizing systems—system optimization may occur through community engagement, advocacy and/or public policy.

Chief medical officers of healthcare organizations, deans and professors at medical schools and other health professions schools, and residency faculty members must take the bold steps of discussing racism, challenging our outdated view of race, and providing adequate resources to remove systemic barriers to health equity. For faculty involved in clinical settings, we must have the expectation that they will work with administrators to measure institutional bias and remove policies that perpetuate these biases. Finally, although most progress towards health equity will require systemic changes, we must also remove people who consciously oppose progress.

The notion that it is possible for someone to have progressed too far in their career to be punished for sociopathic behavior should be a defunct idea. While focusing on system-level issues, the final piece of the puzzle to combating systemic racism is to still hold individuals liable for racist behavior. We should offer opportunities for self-assessment and reflection, encourage diversification of personal networks and interactions, and require that academic departments describe their most critical specialty-specific health disparities with attached action plans on how to look for and address any inequities that exist in their divisions.

KNOWLEDGE, ATTITUDES, AND SKILLS

Knowledge

- Explicit biases are conscious positive or negative feelings about a group of people who share an identity; this includes deliberate preferences for or against these groups.

- Systemic racism—also known as structural racism—is defined as a system of structuring opportunity and assigning value based on the social interpretation of how one looks.

- Systemic racism > Individual racism. Although they might not provoke as much emotion, structural and systemic racism are more damaging on a larger scale than individual acts of racism.

- As discussed with implicit biases, explicit biases that we think of as "positive stereotypes" can still be harmful; this includes harm for group members who do not fit the stereotype or for members of other groups who will be assumed to not possess these positive traits. Furthermore, stereotypes that are based on societal trends or factual data do not consider the systemic inequities that created these differences.

Attitudes

- With regard to systemic racism, intent does not matter! The harmful effects are still the same.

- Focusing too much on individuals (the "bad apples") can create scapegoats and distract us from major systemic issues.

- While changing systems, we still need to hold individuals accountable.

- When we are challenged on our biases, we should embrace them as learning opportunities, not as embarrassing moments. (Try not to be defensive.) For those who teach health equity, be willing to share your own awkward moments that you have experienced.

- Correcting systemic bias must be intentional; structural racism will not be ended with time and patience.

Skills (Explicit Bias)

- Continue frequent self-evaluation to bring implicit biases to the conscious level. Once biases are explicit, remember the bias-reducing strategies of individuating, perspective-taking, and exploring how biases contribute to health disparities in your field.

- Avoid repeated exposure to media and settings that foster or encourage negative stereotypes.

- While being aware of cultural differences and trends, encourage your team to focus on individual patients when providing care.

- To decrease explicit bias at the individual level, structure activities that encourage opportunities for self-assessment and reflection. Implement policies that embrace diversity and encourage interactions between groups.

- Do not just address the individual, instead, create institutional plans that will change the system. (See below.)

Skills (Systemic Racism)

- Use an institutional paradigm—such as those outlined by the AAMC or AAP—to develop meaningful system change and integrate this with your institution's mission.

- Measure institutional bias.

- Establish an organizational consensus on the definitions of race and racism. (The definition of racism should focus on systemic/structural racism.)

- Embrace a paradigm shift that focuses on the social and societal factors that create racial health inequities, as opposed to one that focuses on biological or genetic patterns. (If you are still not convinced of this point, please read Chapter 4 as soon as possible.)

- For those involved in medical education, integrate instruction on achieving health equity from the *onset* of the educational process.

- Require academic departments to identify the top health inequities within their specialty and develop action plans on how to eliminate the associated health disparities.

HOW TO TEACH ABOUT EXPLICIT BIAS

Journalist Juan Williams was fired from National Public Radio (NPR) in 2010 following comments that he made while appearing on the Fox News program *The O'Reilly Factor*.[31] During the segment, he made the following comments:

> *"I'm not a bigot. You know the kind of books I've written about the civil rights movement in this country. But when I get on a plane, I got to tell you, if I see people who are in Muslim garb and I think, you know, they are identifying themselves first and foremost as Muslims, I get worried. I get nervous."*[32]

He justified his fear of Muslims by describing a statement by a "Times Square Bomber" who he reported to have said that Muslims are at war with America. He also inferred that people who disagreed with him were being "politically correct" and were at risk of being "paralyzed" or falling out of touch with "reality." NPR released an official statement that his remarks were "inconsistent with our editorial standards and practices."

These words from Juan Williams are an excellent way to teach about explicit bias, as it demonstrates a public declaration of an admitted bias with an immediate defense of the thought. This was not an implicit bias or unconscious feeling that he could not explain; he knew it and did not think anything was wrong with it. He even preemptively explained that he could not be a bigot because he had written books about the civil rights movement. This same approach is often used when people justify controversial comments about race by pointing towards their volunteer work or by stating that they have Black friends.

Video recordings of Mr. Williams' Fox News interview are available on YouTube or other online video sources for your didactic sessions—these videos will likely still be available by the time of publication of this book, as many of them have been accessible since 2010—and you also have the option of reading his statement above if you do not have audiovisual capabilities.

After playing this video or reading the words of Juan Williams, I recommend first and foremost seeking agreement by the audience that this is a classic example of explicit bias. You can also highlight that while his comments led to his termination and many people referred to them as Islamophobic, he felt that they were appropriate at the time that he made them. Not all explicit biases come from a place of malice, although we have learned by now that intent often does not matter.

Next, ask the audience what they would have done if they had been a supervisor at NPR. This has always resulted in a very lively discussion, and I frequently have to cut off the conversation in the interest of time. Without failure, there are always some participants who agree with firing him, and there are others who feel that he should not have been fired for expressing a genuine fear. I am frequently asked by the audience what I would have done. Here is my response (as with all of my anecdotes, you may feel free to share them with your learners and audiences).

The fear described above was strange to me when I first heard it, as several of my family members are Muslim. Since my childhood, I have been around people whom I love who follow the practices of Islam, and I have never been nervous around women wearing their hijab or men wearing kufi caps. The greeting *As-salamu alaikum* was prominent in the hip hop music that I enjoyed in my childhood. During my freshman year of college, I once supported a friend who was fasting

53

during the month of Ramadan by giving him a bag of post-sunset snacks on a day when he was strapped for cash and the campus cafeteria closed before he could get there.

My first reaction when I heard these words from Juan Williams was one of pity; I felt sorry for him that he had led the kind of life where he ended up afraid of people like some of my friends and family. It was difficult for me to imagine an existence where he had such limited contact with Muslims, as I could not imagine that he had ever spent time with people like my uncle Jamal (R.I.P.), my cousin Waleed, or my college friend Aman. My "punishment" for Mr. Williams might have been to require him to have dinner on a weekly basis with some of my Muslim friends or family—half the time at their house, and half the time at his house. I cannot believe that he would have the same fear by the end of an eight-week stretch of doing this.

At the same time, I do understand that his role as an objective journalist might have been compromised and difficult to continue after his statements, so NPR might have felt that they had no other choice than to terminate him. Also, you have to take my reaction with a grain of salt because I am not a Muslim; I cannot tell Muslim people how they should react to these types of comments. Furthermore, when I imagine someone with a mindset like Juan Williams as a physician at a medical school, I cannot help but think about the damage he could do to Muslim patients, Muslim applicants to the medical school, or Muslim coworkers.

There is one type of potential response to be ready for with this kind of exercise. Although it has only happened rarely with me, I have occasionally had audience participants justify the explicit bias that Juan Williams expressed, even once having someone tell me, "Well it is true that most terrorists are Muslims." During my sessions, I always have audiovisual capabilities, and the screen projector is able to display any internet browser that I open. What I have done when met with these types of comments is to do a simple internet search for some of the mass shootings that have occurred in the United States over the past twenty-five years, stating beforehand that we will look for the first ten results that come up. (I do this in front of everyone, and the first time I did this it was completely spontaneous without knowing what the results would be.)

With little effort, I have found that the killers like the ones at Columbine High School in 1999, the Aurora movie theater in 2012, or the Las Vegas music festival in 2017, are always referred to as "gunmen" or "mass shooters," but never as terrorists.[£] In case anyone is not convinced that these killers would have been referred to as "terrorists" if they had been Muslim, look up the shooters in the 2015 shooting in San Bernardino. At the time that I authored this book, two of the first five results using a common internet search engine referred either to "Islamic terrorism" or "terrorists" for this shooting.

This is an example of how media representations reinforce biases; if a gunman is Muslim, then they are referred to as a terrorist, if they are of any other religion, atheist, or agnostic, then they are referred to as a mass shooter. So, it is not that most terrorists are Muslim, it is just that our media tends to only call shooters terrorists if they are Muslim. A separate component of this health equity curriculum addresses religious intolerance—presented in Chapter 7 in this book—but this is a valuable discussion for this unit, and you should definitely counter any religious biases that come out during this activity instead of waiting for the session on religion.

HOW TO TEACH ABOUT SYSTEMIC RACISM

This chapter discusses the importance of countering individual biases but also discussing systemic issues. Therefore, I also recommend supplementing the explicit bias exercise above with an example of systemic racism. I again propose playing a short video clip—available on YouTube for the past five years and included in this chapter's references—this time of Paul LePage, the former governor of Maine. In January 2016, he was discussing a bill that he wanted introduced into law to address the drug problem in his state. During this press conference, he said the following:

"...the traffickers...are guys that are named 'D-Money,' 'Smoothie,' 'Shiftee,' these type of guys. They come from Connecticut and New York,...sell their heroin...and...impregnate a young White girl before they leave..."[33]

Ask your audience who they think he was referring to with these nicknames, and what image he is portraying when discussing White girls being impregnated. I have universally received the response that he is using euphemisms for young African American men and that he is invoking a stereotypical image of predatory Black males. Even if your group does not agree that these are veiled racist words, it does not matter; this is more of a discussion on *systemic* racism, not a debate about whether the former governor is a racist. (Remember I told you that it is futile to discuss this anyway.) To segue into the discussion on systemic racism, finish with these additional comments from Paul LePage regarding his war on drugs:

"When you go to war, if you know the enemy and the enemy dresses in red and you dress in blue, then you shoot at red. You shoot at the enemy. You try to identify the enemy and the enemy right now, the overwhelming majority of people coming in, are people of color or people of Hispanic origin."

The twist in the story that you are going to present to your audience is that the crime statistics from the Federal Bureau of Investigation (FBI) completely contradict what Paul LePage said.[34] He doubled down on his claim that "the overwhelming majority" of drug dealers were "people of color or people of Hispanic origin" by saying that "90-plus percent" of arrests for heroin trafficking were Black and Hispanic men. In the state of Maine in 2014, Black people only accounted for 14 percent of a total of 1,211 drug sale and manufacturing arrests, and they accounted for just 7.4 percent of 5,791 total drug arrests. (Spoiler alert: arrests involving Hispanic men did not bring these 14 percent and 7 percent totals up anywhere close to 90 percent, or even close to 25 percent for that matter.)

He made his comments at the beginning of 2016, and the FBI had not released data for 2015 yet. Maine's Department of Public Safety does not include race and ethnicity when reporting or analyzing crime, so the then governor's comments were completely made up and not based on any factual information. He encouraged citizens who have concealed carrying permits to load up their guns and help "get rid of the drug dealers."[35]

In closing, ask your participants about the *system* that is likely created by this governor who also recommended using the National Guard to fight drug trafficking.[36] Have them imagine being a Black or Latino man pulled over by the police in Maine; then ask them to imagine how much worse this experience would be if they have a New York or Connecticut license plate tag. Even if individual police officers do not have explicit biases or racist thoughts against African American or Hispanic men, imagine the implicit thoughts in their minds when the highest elected official in the state has repeatedly referred to these men as an enemy that needs to be shot and killed.

These same implicit and explicit biases would likely also be present in jurors or judges who preside over the few Black and Latino men who are arrested and tried in drug arrests. (They might also be present in vigilante citizens who follow their governor's edict to help them get rid of drug dealers with their personal guns.) This exemplifies why individual behavior should not be excused, as people in positions of power can cause even more injustice in systems that are already structurally racist.

To drive home the definitions of systemic racism and mechanisms for combating it, here are two questions that were used for a recent CME event that I provided for a state chapter of the American Academy of Pediatrics. The answers are in bold, and you can feel free to use or modify them.

1. Systemic racism is defined as:

    a. A belief that a certain group is inherently inferior to another group, whereas others are inherently superior

b. The presence of racist people in the leadership structure of healthcare systems

c. A system of structuring opportunity and assigning value based on the social interpretation of how one looks

d. Hatred for groups of people based on their race

2. Ways to combat racism in healthcare include all of the following *except*:

a. Measuring institutional bias

b. Coming to a consensus on how we define race and racism

c. Addressing both individual biases and problems in our healthcare systems

d. Researching genetic causes of racial and ethnic health disparities

e. Promoting a diverse work environment

£Please see footnote in Notes for comment regarding references for internet search on recent mass shooters.

CHAPTER 4

RACE-BASED MEDICAL DECISION-MAKING

DR. BONZO'S BUNGLE OF THE MONTH:
Failure to Build Coalitions

My almost-twenty years as an attending physician have exposed me to easily over a thousand resident physicians and medical students who trained at several different medical schools and residency programs. One thing that I noticed early in my career was that some of my learners' clinical presentations always began with three routine pieces of patient information: age, gender, and race. Two (personal) details of my life made this inclusion of race an odd occurrence for me. First, growing up as a Black male in Georgia—including being called "the n- word" for the first time by a classmate at age seven—exposed me to incidents of racism that undoubtedly made me hyperaware of mentions of race later in life. Second, my time at a Historically Black College and University (HBCU) for my undergraduate and medical school education led to training that deemphasized the importance of race in medical decision-making.

While race and ethnicity were sometimes considered to be important aspects of the social history, we were never taught that they needed to be included in the introductory sentence of every single patient presentation. This was in direct contrast to the presentations I heard later in life that regularly considered race to be as important as a patient's age or sex in treating all patients. For these presentations that uniformly included race, no other aspect of the social history (e.g., smoking status) was used for all presentations.

In discussions with multiple medical students and resident physicians, many of them stated that they felt race was important in medical decision-making, specifically when it comes to the diagnosis of genetic disorders and making decisions about pharmacotherapy. After probing for examples, the most common responses were the selection of antihypertensive medication and the strong association between sickle cell disease and the Black race. Beyond that, students were unable to explain why they begin their presentations with, "This is a forty-three-year-old *African American* male..." when the patient was presenting with something else like a sprained ankle.

In the "Pre-2020" section of the Preface, I mentioned my graduate school interdisciplinary training in health disparities. During this time, I met evolutionary biologist Dr. Joseph Graves, who was gracious enough to send me two of his books and who strongly challenged the idea that race had a consistent or reliable genetic pattern. After reading his books, I became convinced for good that race is a social construct and that viewing it as a biological construct distracts from the social factors that create disparities between races. With additional research and exploration over time this message was solidified for me, and I made it a mission of mine to eliminate the practice of race-based medicine in the clinical and academic settings in which I worked.

Closely related, I also desired to eliminate race from the opening line of our learners' clinical presentations and put it back in the social history where it belongs. Unfortunately, as a young instructor, and later assistant professor, I did not have the voice or access to audiences that wielded the power to assist me with this goal.

I presented my thoughts on race-based medicine in various settings—as the keynote speaker for our medical school's Student National Medical Association (SNMA) Fall Affair in 2010, and during an oral presentation at the Society of Teachers of Family Medicine (STFM) Medical Education Conference in Long Beach, California, in 2012. When I was promoted to associate professor and became the associate dean of diversity, equity, and inclusion at my medical school in 2015, I finally seized the opportunity to move beyond talking about this and more towards action.

I took my message to the curriculum committee of my medical school as one of my first orders of business, with a request to have our students eliminate non-pertinent mentions of race in clinical presentations, to revise our student cases to eliminate racial stereotypes, and to shift the paradigm from race-based medicine to a social view of race. Ahead of my meeting with the curriculum committee, I sent out a short (less than four pages) article for pre-reading from the journal *Family Medicine* entitled, "The Role of Race in the Clinical Presentation," by physician Matthew Anderson and colleagues.[1] I was excited for one of my first opportunities to help create systemic change.

When I was called upon to present my information at the meeting, I began to rattle off my list of demands as described above, and I immediately noticed the stunned looks on everyone's faces. These looks were followed in short order by questions from committee members who were skeptical about what I was saying. I was asked the question that is still to this day the most common one that I receive on this topic: "What about sickle cell disease?" They asked me about several things that were addressed in the pre-reading, so I finally asked how many people had a chance to read the article. To my disappointment, not a single person had read the article. (Not one!) This was very frustrating, and I expressed amazement that people were arguing with me on a topic they had not researched themselves.

One of the committee members asked me for more data, and I responded, "There is this great thing called the internet, and it has all the data that you need." I was condescending on purpose for the remainder of the meeting, and there were no changes made at that time or for years to come. In fact, it would be another five years before my medical school made these changes to our curriculum.

This bungle of the month is different from the previous ones in that I did not have an unconscious bias against anyone, and I did not stereotype anybody. I was actually presenting accurate information that would promote health equity, but the bungle was in my approach to creating systemic change. I botched the meeting by leading with the requests before explaining the evidence behind them. I assumed that people would read the materials ahead of time and I did not have a contingency plan to bring people up to speed if they did not. I also allowed my disappointment to turn into irritation, which interfered with my goal despite perhaps being justified to some degree. The narrative of the meeting turned into Dr. Bonzo arguing with everyone about race and chastising them for not having time in their busy schedules to read his article.

My frustration led me to table my plans for eliminating race-based medicine and instead focus on other issues: creating an inclusive environment in our medical school, reinvigorating our SNMA chapters, increasing collaboration between our student diversity groups, developing pipelines with HBCUs, and developing a mentorship program for URM students. I also avoided the curriculum committee and focused on taking my messages about race and ethnicity outside of my institutional walls.

What I did not realize until later was that the setting of that curriculum meeting was an ideal one that I did not take advantage of. With a group that was inexperienced in this topic, it was an ideal opportunity to use my personal teaching style to present the information in a simple, enthusiastic, and entertaining format using a "health equity lens." The health equity lens starts with the mission of the institution and then aligns policies and research with the health equity principles that you are presenting,[2] similar to the theme of the AAMC Institutional Diversity Paradigm discussed in the previous chapter.

It would have grabbed everyone's attention if I had led with our school's mission and explained that the group that sponsors our accrediting body recommends a specific paradigm to achieve our mission. I could have then used the techniques that I describe later in this chapter to define race and ethnicity, explain how they are currently used in the practice of medicine, discuss the poor-quality evidence that led to these practices, and then present information about the harms of using a biological view of race and ethnicity.

Spoiler alert: this is the exact approach that I used in 2020, and this time around the result was a friendly, non-contentious, hour-long meeting that accomplished all of the goals that I had failed to meet in the original meeting five years earlier.

DEFINITIONS

At the heart of the decision to begin all patient presentations with the race or ethnicity of a patient is the suggestion that there is a biological or genetic component to these demographic categories. As discussed in Chapter 1, there are obvious trends that demonstrate a link between race, ethnicity, and certain health outcomes. These trends do not, however, clarify whether the differences that we see for the health outcomes are driven by innate biological differences between races, social factors, or a combination of both. Before we discuss this, let us again start by clarifying the definitions of some of the terms that I have referenced.

The *social determinants of health* are the non-biomedical factors that influence health outcomes, such as poverty, adequacy of housing, income level, access to employment, exposure to stress or violence, and socioeconomic status.[3] Chapter 9 of this book discusses the social determinants of health in detail, and it explains that social, environmental, and economic factors have a much greater effect on health than clinical care. The World Health Organization (WHO) concurs that social determinants are the "single most important determinant of one's health status."[4] However, even if we agree that social determinants have a greater impact on health compared to biological determinants, the question still remains whether racial and ethnic categories have a legitimate biological or genetic origin.

The United States (U.S.) Census Bureau and Office of Management and Budget (OMB) have traditionally recognized a minimum of five major racial categories:[5,6]

1. White (referred to as Caucasian by some, although this term is falling out of favor)

2. Black/African American

3. American Indian/Alaska Native (also known as Native American or, in Canada, as First Nations)

4. Asian

5. Native Hawaiian/Pacific Islander

People may identify as more than one race, although the percentage of people who do so is extremely low. Within the five major race classifications, a person can choose any of several more specific classifications. For example, people who identify as Asian can specify if they are Asian Indian/South Indian, Chinese, Filipino, Korean, Japanese, Vietnamese, or Other Asian. Similarly, Native Hawaiian/Pacific Islanders may specifically identify as descending from the native people of Hawaii, Guam, Samoa, etc. Members of a racial group "have origins in any of the original peoples" of various countries or locations that the racial groups are traditionally identified with. When people do not know the origins of their ancestors—as is the case with many Black Americans because of the institution of slavery in the United States—then they are often assigned a race based on phenotypic physical features that are stereotypical of specific races.

Until recently, the U.S. Census Bureau has recognized only two ethnic categories:

1. Hispanic/Latino (see Footnote #1 in the Preface for additional comments on use of Latino/a/x)
2. Not Hispanic or Latino

Although discussions of race often include Latin American people as a race, they are technically an ethnic group. Although people can identify with more than one racial category, they have historically only been allowed to choose one ethnicity. Therefore, it is possible for a biracial individual to identify as Black and White; it is also possible for Hispanic people to identify as either Black, White, or both (or any other race for that matter).

There are significant inconsistencies in the tracking of data about race and ethnicity that expose the flaws in their definitions and categorizations.[7] Race is subjective, social, political, and fluid over time. Carolyn Klatt (a librarian colleague of mine) once pointed out that sometime between 1988 and 1990, former president Barack Obama—who had a White mother and Black father—would have changed from being Black to being White according to the National Center for Health Statistics. Prior to 1989, a person's race was considered to be the same as that of their non-White parent. But after 1989, it was assigned as the same race of the mother on their birth certificate. In recent years, the standard has changed again to one of "self-identified race," in which the person chooses the race that they identify as. That means Barack Obama was Black again in time to become the first African American president of the United States.

THE FALLACIES AND DANGERS OF RACE-BASED MEDICAL DECISION-MAKING

Race does not have a biological definition, but rather a political and social one that is fluid and changes over time independent of scientific discovery. Nevertheless, the medical community uses race as a scientific variable in several prominent clinical situations: calculation of atherosclerotic cardiovascular disease (ASCVD) risk, calculation of glomerular filtration rate (GFR), decisions on pharmacotherapy for hypertension, and interpretation of pulmonary function testing. These diagnostic and clinical predictor tools do not include the social and environmental factors that influence racial differences in health outcomes. Furthermore, they do not highlight the potentially harmful effects of using race to make medical decisions. Although we may hear about biological or genetic differences between races, there is more variation *within* races than there is *between* them.[8]

When using identical blood pressure and lipid data in the Pooled Cohort ASCVD Calculator, a forty-year-old White male smoker has a lower cardiovascular risk than a forty-year-old Black male non-smoker. Without considering lifestyle, drug use, or the significant heterogeneity in the African American population, this decision-making tool lumps all Black people together. The guidelines from the Joint National Committee (JNC) on the management of high blood pressure recommend against using monotherapy with angiotensin-converting enzyme inhibitors (ACEIs) in the treatment of hypertension in African American patients.[9] This recommendation was heavily influenced by the findings of the Antihypertensive and Lipid-Lowering Treatment to Prevent Heart Attack Trial (ALLHAT), which showed worse cardiovascular outcomes for Black patients treated with lisinopril.[10] Unfortunately, this is sometimes translated into the idea that "ACEIs do not work in Black people," despite the fact that these questionable racial differences are not seen in patients treated with combination therapy.[11,12]

Even taken at face value, a racial difference in the efficacy of ACEI monotherapy is explained by social factors, not genetic causes. More than a decade ago, the American Heart Association published a report from the International Society on Hypertension in Blacks that linked poor blood pressure control in Black patients to non-physiologic factors such as high stress levels, less physical activity, higher rates of obesity, and low-potassium diets.[13] Racial differences in renin-angiotensin activity resolve when Black patients decrease sodium intake, and there is more variation in renin-angiotensin activity within the Black race than there is when comparing Black and White people. Treating Black patients as a monolithic group stereotypes them without considering that they are not all obese, and many follow the DASH diet and exercise regularly.

Despite having worse outcomes for chronic kidney disease (CKD), race-based equations assign a higher GFR—i.e., better kidney function—for Black patients with the same creatinine value as people of other races. This is based on questionable racial differences related to appendicular skeletal muscle mass, bone density, and markers of nutritional status (e.g., albumin).[14-16] As is the case with hypertension, these racial differences are often presented without considering non-biological causes and without considering the significant variation within individual races. The result is that a creatinine value of 1.59 is "normal" for a Black male (GFR > 60), but consistent with stage 3 CKD for a White male (GFR 52). Whenever GFR values fall near the cutoffs between stages of CKD, White patients receive more aggressive recommendations while Black patients receive more conservative interventions.

Peralta et al. asserted that the use of race-based GFR equations has been shown to "systematically miss a high-risk group of Blacks at a time in the disease course when interventions are crucial."[17] By inflating their GFR, it leads to underdiagnosis of CKD in Black patients, makes them less likely to be referred to a nephrologist, and also makes them less likely to be eligible for kidney transplantation. Additionally, the beliefs about the use of ACEIs in Black patients mentioned above can prevent African Americans with CKD from receiving one of the key medications that can prevent progression of their kidney disease.

Race is a sloppy, inconsistent proxy for genetics and biology, and we should move towards eliminating it from medical decision-making. This includes reconsidering our use of race in clinical decision-making tools such as the calculator for the likelihood of a successful vaginal birth after cesarean (VBAC) delivery.[18] In a country where Black women have significantly higher maternal morbidity and mortality, this calculator assigns a lower chance of VBAC success for them compared to White women or non-Black Hispanic women. Instead of encouraging a mode of delivery that can improve recovery time and lower the risk of infection or postpartum hemorrhage, this calculator potentially discourages obstetric providers from offering Black women a trial of labor after a cesarean section. Instead of treating Black women as a homogeneous group, we should be aggressively studying the social and systemic factors that have historically resulted in more cesarean sections.

While the VBAC and ASCVD calculators typically assign higher risk to African Americans, the Fractured Risk Assessment Tool (FRAX) for estimating osteoporotic fracture risk behaves like the GFR equation and results in a lower risk assessment for Black patients.[19] In general, FRAX assigns a ten-year fracture risk to non-White women that is approximately half the risk for White women. Black women are less likely to be screened for osteoporosis, less likely to be treated for osteoporosis, less likely to receive a dual-energy X-ray absorptiometry (DXA) scan following a hip fracture, and more likely to die or become disabled following a hip fracture. Yet we systematically assign a lower fracture risk to the entire Black community without considering how diverse that community is.

For all the calculators and predictor tools mentioned, none of them provide any scientific rationale about what race to input if a patient has one Black parent and one White parent. There are almost no other aspects of the practice of medicine that result in such dramatic differences in medical management—whether to use a statin or

ACEI, whether someone is diagnosed with obstructive lung disease, or whether someone receives a kidney transplant—simply based on a patient's subjective report about their identity.

We should focus on the social factors that create the differences that we see between races, and we should also discuss how to screen for these social factors and behaviors instead of assuming things about people based on their skin color. The rigor that is demanded in evidence-based medicine often eludes studies of race, as exemplified by the studies that led to the Black and Asian correction factors for pulmonary function testing.[20-21] A systematic review of spirometry—spirometers being the devices that measure lung function—revealed that only 17.3 percent of studies actually defined race and/or ethnicity, and 94 percent of articles failed to examine socioeconomic status as a potential confounder.[22]

The idea of physiological differences between the lungs of Black and White people dates back to the days of chattel slavery in the United States. Dr. Samuel Cartwright, inventor of one of the first spirometers, did not consider that it was the squalor and disease that enslaved Africans lived amongst that caused any racial differences in pulmonary function; he assumed that the differences were due to inferior genetics.[23] Then again, this is the same man who thought that the desire to escape slavery was a mental illness that some Black people suffered from, and that the first-line treatment for this disorder was corporal punishment.

Race-based approaches to medicine reinforce a system that assumes biological causes of health inequities, which can cause us to ignore the social determinants of health that are the true drivers for racial disparities in health outcomes. This creates a racist system that withholds organ transplants and preventive services from Black patients with CKD, withholds ACEIs from Black patients that might benefit from them, and ignores the social or environmental factors that cause differences in the lung function of Black and Asian people. As family physicians, we should inform patients of the limitations when we use race-based algorithms, and we should look for social explanations to racial/ethnic disparities. As we continue to improve the ways in which we competently address social determinants, we should be proud to join the ranks of the American Medical Association, the American Academy of Family Physicians, and other organizations who, once and for all, declare race as a social construct instead of a biological one.[24,25]

KNOWLEDGE, ATTITUDES, AND SKILLS

Knowledge

Race-based medicine causes us to do the following:

- Ignore the social determinants of cardiovascular health for Black/African American patients (e.g., tendency to prescribe a statin for higher heart disease risk instead of addressing the underlying causes of diet, exercise, and stress).

- Withhold lifesaving and kidney-saving medications from Black patients with diabetes mellitus and hypertension.

- Delay initiation of angiotensin converting enzyme inhibitor (ACE-I) or angiotensin receptor blocker (ARB) therapy for Black patients with chronic kidney disease.

- Delay referrals to nephrology/kidney specialists for Black patients.

- Withhold kidney transplants for Black patients with end-stage renal disease.

- Tell patients with chronic obstructive pulmonary disease (COPD) that their lungs are normal because they are Black or Asian.

- Ignore the social and environmental factors in lung disease.

Attitudes

- Race-based medical decision-making and a social determinants of health approach to health care are diametrically opposed.

69

- Racial, ethnic, and cultural factors are often important components of patient context, but they should almost *never* be used for medical decision-making.

- Paradoxically, while rethinking race-based medicine, we can use biological determinants of health to reinforce the importance of social determinants of health (i.e., describe trends in health disparities between races, but then explain the underlying social causes).

Skills

- When you see racial and ethnic disparities and inequities, look for SOCIAL explanations (i.e., social determinants of health).

- For cardiovascular disease, focus on:

  1. Treating each person like an individual.

  2. Diet and exercise (lifestyle) for all patients.

  3. Centering new research on stress, racism, and allostatic load instead of tenuous genetic differences between races.

- For hypertension, focus on:

  1. Lifestyle changes to decrease health disparities in the treatment of hypertension (less focus on which medication to prescribe for which race).

  2. Community-level interventions to increase physical activity.

  3. Community-level interventions to address food insecurity or access to healthy foods.

- For kidney disease, focus on:

  1. Continuing the trend of getting rid of race-based GFR equations.

  2. The aforementioned interventions for reducing disparities in hypertension.

3. The social factors that lead to health inequities for diabetes mellitus.

- For obstructive lung disease, focus on:

1. Social and environmental factors that lead to lung disease.

2. Environmental justice initiatives to decrease pollution, overcrowding, and the high prevalence of allergens in some public housing.

- For *all* medical conditions, focus on increasing access to high-quality health care for all people.

HOW TO TEACH ABOUT THE LIMITATIONS OF RACE-BASED MEDICINE

Cardiovascular Disease Risk Case

Along with the implicit bias exercise described in Chapter 2, this is one of the exercises that has garnered the most attention whenever I share it during invited lectures and didactic sessions. For this session, take a look at the example of the American Heart Association (AHA) and American College of Cardiology (ACC) consensus guidelines from a few years ago, which recommended the use of a pooled cohort calculator to estimate a person's atherosclerotic cardiovascular disease (ASCVD) risk. In doing so, we input data about a person—their age, sex assigned at birth, blood pressure values, whether they have diabetes, and of course their race—and this calculator estimates that person's ten-year risk of developing heart disease.

When I turned forty years old more than a half-decade ago, I performed this calculation on myself following my annual physical. I was pleased with the objective findings of my visit:

- blood pressure: 118/80, pulse: 58
- body mass index (BMI): 23.29 kg/m^2
- total cholesterol: 183, HDL cholesterol: 81, LDL cholesterol: 85
- fasting glucose (blood sugar): 80

Using the AHA/ACC ASCVD risk calculator, my physician told me that my estimated ten-year cardiac risk was 2.3 percent. *Not bad*, I thought to myself, *that is a 97.7 percent chance that I'll make it to age fifty with no heart disease.* At the same time, I also wondered what my risk would be if you made me a White man. So, I changed my race to White on the calculator, left all the other demographic and health information the same, and my risk dropped from 2.3 percent to 0.4 percent. Almost a six-fold decrease. Curiosity got the best of me, so I just had to figure out what Asian Bonzo's risk was. After changing my race to Asian, I received the same result that White Bonzo had—0.4 percent (Image 5).

That was the moment I realized for the first time—after using this calculator in my clinical practice for years—that if you input any race besides Black, you will receive the same result. This clinical decision-making tool used by physicians all over the country was essentially telling me that Black people are uniquely different from everyone else on the planet, while all other races share similar, uniform heart disease risks.

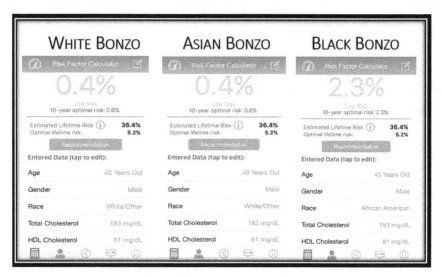

As the rabbit hole opened up, I randomly changed the data to see what my estimated heart disease risk would be if I made certain changes about myself. I was disappointed that Black Bonzo always seemed to have the higher risk, even when White or Asian Bonzo's blood pressure is higher, or cholesterol is worse. For example, if I gave my hypothetical White Bonzo a case of prehypertension, prediabetes, high LDL and total cholesterol, and low HDL cholesterol (which is a negative risk factor for heart disease), his risk was still lower than his Black alter ego. In this imaginary world, I also envisioned him being an obese, sedentary individual with a somewhat high resting heart rate; this gentleman also seldom exercised and never ate any vegetables, but none of these affected his risk as much as race did. Here are his stats:

- blood pressure: 131/81, pulse: 86
- body mass index (BMI): 30.1 kg/m^2
- total cholesterol: 203, HDL cholesterol: 39, LDL cholesterol: 126
- fasting glucose: 101

Despite these worsening blood pressure, blood sugar, and cholesterol values, the ASCVD risk calculation for this person is only 1.7 percent when their race is White, which is still lower than the 2.3 percent risk for the real Bonzo who had more ideal vital sign and laboratory data. So finally, the payoff. I pulled up the original White Bonzo again—he of the lowly 0.4 percent heart disease risk—and made him a smoker. *Ha! That'll show him!* I thought. *There's no way his risk is lower than mine now.* I was stunned that White Bonzo's heart disease risk was still lower at 1.3 percent—even after you made him a smoker—compared to Black, non-smoking Bonzo whose risk is still at 2.3 percent (Image 6). Yes, you heard me correctly, people…*being Black is more dangerous than smoking*!

So, we have a medical decision-making tool that comments on my health and future health-related risks based on my self-identified race. It does not consider how much I exercise, if I abuse drugs, whether I live a sedentary lifestyle, or how much stress I have in my life. Interestingly, this tool is based on population level information and statistics, so to some degree it is based on objective data. However, it does not appreciate the fact that racial categories are extremely heterogeneous, and that there is more variation *within* races than there is *between* races. (If that seems confusing to anyone, then the next recommended exercise below will help to clarify this for your audience.)

At the same time, the fact that the population level data has demonstrated results that lead to this kind of a calculator is a significant indictment of our society that the social experience of being Black for many people is more dangerous than smoking cigarettes.

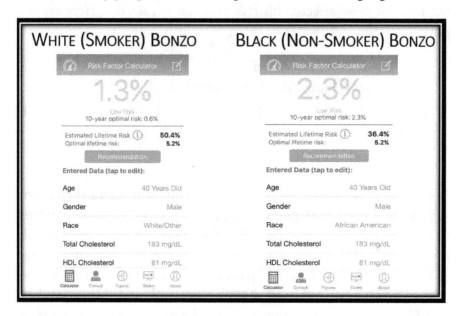

MORE VARIATION WITHIN RACES AND ETHNICITIES THAN BETWEEN THEM

While debating the existence of a genetic pattern to race, one of my medical students brought up the "fact" that Asian people have higher rates of gastric (or stomach) cancer. I looked up data from the International Agency for Research on Cancer (IARC) and the International Association of Cancer Registries,[26] and then I graphed out the results for the incidences of stomach cancer. I also compared the gastric cancer rates between countries based on sex assigned at birth (reported by the IARC at the time of publication in a binary fashion as either male or female). I found that two East Asian countries, Japan and Korea, have by far the highest rates of gastric cancer on the planet; however, other East Asian countries like the Philippines and Thailand have some of the *lowest* rates on the plane with a risk similar to White Americans.

Based on the graph in Image 7, you could say that, compared to Black Americans like me, Asian males have a *lower* risk of stomach cancer. This would be considered accurate based on this data if the Asian males that you are referencing are Filipino or Thai, for example. Conversely, you might also be telling the truth if you said that they have a *higher* risk of stomach cancer compared to Black males in America, if the Asian people you are referring to are predominantly Japanese or Korean. These racial categories, such as "Asian," do not consider the significant variation that exists within the race and the associated countries of origin.

In the end, someone from Japan might be more genetically different from someone in Thailand than they are from an African American. Racial data often inadvertently presents an incomplete or inaccurate picture based on the subgroups that are included. More concerning is that racial data can be manipulated to present a story that fits whatever narrative the manipulator wants to present.

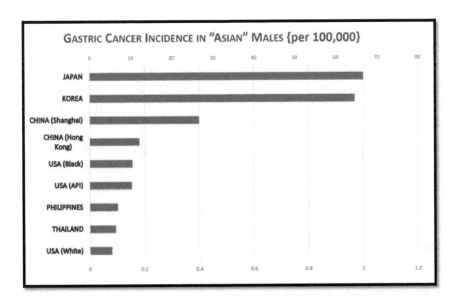

One unique characteristic of the Black race is that, because of the history of slavery in this country, we typically do not know the ancestral countries of origin of most US-born Black Americans. So, unlike the example I just presented for stomach cancer, I cannot give you a breakdown of American-born Black people stratified by the countries of origin of their ancestors. Now, you may be saying, "Well at least we can do this for other races besides Black people," but…not so fast! If you further breakdown the stomach cancer stats from earlier by country, you will see more variation *within* countries like China than *between* China and other countries. (Noticing a similar theme yet?)

There is more of a gap between the cancer rates in Shanghai and Hong Kong (more than a two-fold difference) than there is between Hong Kong and the African American population. So, remember there was more of a difference between Japanese and Filipino males than there was between Asian and African American males? Or more difference between the incidence rates in Korea and Thailand than there was between the rates among Asian males and White American males collectively? You will often see the same thing the more you break down groups within a specific country, within a state, within a city, within a zip code, and so on.

The same heterogeneity seen with racial categorizations occurs when grouping people by ethnicity, as seen on the graph in Image 8. Using Hispanic or Latino ethnicity (again based on sex assigned at birth), certain Latin American countries have very high rates of gastric cancer among males while others have very low rates. The rates in Costa Rica and Colombia are higher than the rates in some areas of China, while countries like Cuba have rates that are lower than the ones seen in the United States. The Hispanic stomach cancer data also demonstrates two very interesting points that cause a genetic theory of race and ethnicity to further lose credibility for one common reason.

First, notice that countries like Cuba that are geographically close to the United States have rates that are similar to those seen in the US. This raises the question about whether the variation in cancer rates is related more to the physical environment and less to the genetics of the people inhabiting those areas. Second, notice that Hispanic males

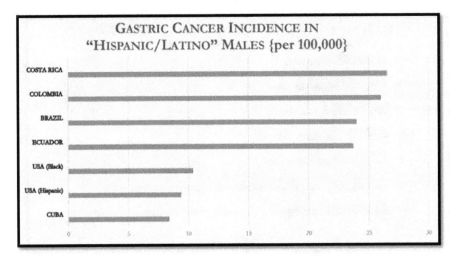

living in the United States have rates that are even lower than African American men. This again suggests that environmental explanations exist, given that the stomach cancer risk decreases for many Hispanic groups after they move to this country. If Costa Ricans had a genetic predisposition to gastric cancer at birth, then this increased risk should not go away just from moving to a new country.

One more complicating factor for racial and ethnic trends in disease incidence occurs when adding the variable of sex. In all of the countries that I analyzed, males had much higher rates of gastric cancer compared to females from the same nation. This demonstrates that analyses of race and ethnicity can easily be skewed one way or the other depending on the number of males versus females in the studies. Data from the graph in Image 9 shows that there is a higher rate of gastric cancer among Iranian males than among Japanese females, even though overall Japan has the highest incidence in the world when combining males and females. If we believe in a genetic or physiological basis for these disparities, then it would be easy to ignore unequal distribution of sex or gender in studies of race and ethnicity.

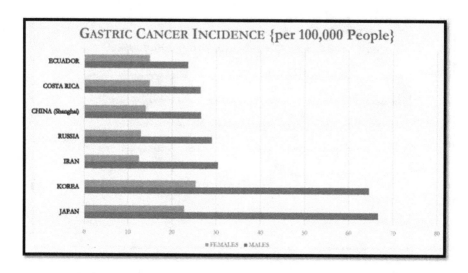

In closing, let us summarize why being Black is more dangerous than smoking if there is not a genetic reason. The answer boils down to the social determinants of health, which we alluded to earlier in this chapter and which we will explore in depth in Chapter 9. The social experience of being Black is what causes the differences between the large racial groups—one way to translate this is that racism is the risk factor, not race. The problem is, we have no way to measure what factors affect which people, and to what extent (think again about our discussions on intersectionality in the Preface and Chapter 1) which limits the generalizability of any race-based calculators.

Using the example from earlier in this chapter, the International Society on Hypertension in Blacks reported more than a decade ago that the blood pressure differences between African Americans and other groups are related to non-genetic factors, and even the physiological differences that we see are caused by social factors such as a tendency towards higher-calorie diets and a life with more daily stress.[13] Although these are general trends, lumping all Black people together makes assumptions about us—a.k.a. stereotyping—without considering the Black yogi, Black vegan, or Black marathon runner. (And yes, I realize I just stereotyped yogis; I'm sure that some of them are stressed out too.)

CHAPTER 5

SEXISM IN MEDICINE

> ### DR. BONZO'S BUNGLE OF THE MONTH:
> #### The Angry Woman Trope

Women physicians who I have worked with have told me about their frustrations in the medical field where they are frequently assumed to be the nurse instead of the doctor, even when they wear a long white coat or when their name badge says "MD" or "DO." They have pointed out the times when patients would prefer to hear advice from male medical students rather than from female chief residents or attending physicians.

I used to rationalize or explain away these occurrences until one of my friends accurately pointed out that the clinic staff always referred to her by her first name but called me Dr. Reddick or Dr. Bonzo. (They also called the other men "Doctor.") At the end of Chapter 2, I described how my own implicit bias sometimes leads me to assume that a physician that I hear about is a man. It rarely happens anymore now that I am aware of it, especially since I now recognize it as a bigger deal than I once thought. (More on that in a moment.)

I have had other implicit biases that have been brought to the conscious level, including one involving women sportscasters. One day while watching a professional basketball game with friends, I mentioned that I was not a big fan of sports broadcaster Doris Burke, and the group around me was stunned. I complained that she appeared to be bored while announcing National Basketball Association (NBA) games. One guy grabbed his phone and pulled up a YouTube video of her dribbling a basketball between her legs while holding a clipboard and wearing high heels. He was having a hard time accepting Doris Burke as "boring" as he followed up with another video of her joking around with celebrities in the crowd.

I think my brain tried to move towards the "angry woman" trope; I stated that I seemed to remember her having contentious interviews with players, although I could not recall the details. One person in the group had a bit of a journalism background, and they mentioned that women who cover men's sports are often sexually harassed, they are sometimes purposefully excluded or have their access to athletes limited, and they at times are not taken seriously if they do not present themselves in a certain way. They mentioned that those episodes I was vaguely recalling probably had some context to them based on the systemic issues that women like Doris Burke face on a daily basis.

I have always been disgusted with men who make misogynistic comments against women involved in sports, and I have been a fan of several great women sports' reporters and journalists such as Linda Cohn and Jemele Hill. As I tried to justify my criticism of Doris Burke, I realized that I was sounding a lot like the people who declare that they can't be racist because they voted for Barack Obama. I did some reflection and realized that I did not necessarily have a bias against women reporters, but I did have the bias of preferring the ones who always maintained a cheerful persona...as if they were there to entertain me and not to do their job.

Interestingly, from that day on, I was never able to witness any of these alleged boring Doris Burke moments. I only saw a sportscaster who had an even mix of humor, supreme basketball knowledge, and assertiveness when people tried to dodge or challenge her questions. Needless to say, I am now a big Doris Burke fan.

Unfortunately, these instances of implicit bias pale in comparison to my bungle of the month, which occurred in 2017—at a health equity summit no less! As one of the organizers of the summit, I had the pleasure of meeting one of our speakers who at the time had recently been named as the chancellor at a major university. She described the challenges women face in obtaining mentorship during medical training and in academic medical careers. One barrier that she described was a fear by would-be male mentors that they will be falsely accused of sexual harassment if they have an unwitnessed meeting with a female mentee. She explained that some men follow the Billy

Graham Rule, whereby they will not meet alone with a woman who is not a family member as a means of avoiding sexual temptation or false accusations.[1]

During the summit, I mentioned my specific interest in increasing the number of Black men in medicine following the AAMC's 2015 report, *Altering the Course*.[2] The speaker was supportive of these types of efforts, and she asked others to ensure that we also do not forget about Black women. She asked if I had heard concerns from men who follow guidelines such as the Billy Graham Rule or if I had similar worries. When I told her that I did not have a lot of concerns, but I did typically keep the door open whenever meeting with a woman alone, she gave me a look that I still remember to this day. She replied, "That's…interesting," and proceeded with her presentation. I could sense that she had an issue with my response, so I carved out some time to meet with her afterwards. Someone else approached her at the same time and she quickly waived them off and said, "Can we chat later? I have some mentoring to do."

The speaker mentioned that there was a systemic inequity that I created by giving men a safe, confidential meeting environment without providing the same opportunity for women. This could make women less likely to be open about their concerns, needs, or struggles out of fear that someone might walk by an open door and hear them while they are talking. I told her about an instance in the remote past that rattled me and likely influenced my behavior.

Years ago, a group of my students asked what I was doing over the weekend, and I mentioned that I was going to be completely lazy and do nothing because my wife was out of town. One of the women in the group stayed behind and asked me if I wanted to hang out over the weekend. I felt uneasy and told her that was not appropriate as her teacher, to which she replied that she promised she would not tell anyone. To this day, I do not know if she was making a pass at me or just trying to be friendly with a younger faculty member, but my mind started racing with anxiety as I again declined her invitation.

I started to wonder if she would perceive this as rejection and become upset, or if she might tell people that I was the one who asked her out to try and head off any awkwardness if I retold the story. The student appeared a little embarrassed, but her demeanor did not change for the remainder of the academic year. I concluded that I had dodged a bullet and decided that I needed to carry myself differently so that I did not give people the wrong idea, lead people on, or create a physical environment that would allow this kind of thing to happen again in the future; hence, my "open door policy" and other related behaviors.

The speaker was not impressed by my story. She asked me to retell my story but replace "women" with "Black men." I did not carry out her request, because I was immediately embarrassed by the idea of someone saying, "I always keep the door open when meeting with Black men because I think one of them tried to hit on me back in the day." She explained that I was stereotyping young women as "vixens" who were trying to seduce their professor. Putting aside how incredibly low the incidence of false accusations actually is, punishing the entire group because of the behavior of one or a few members perpetuates bias and inequity.

Since that conversation, I have tried to treat all mentees the same and have provided mentorship to men, women, and people of any gender. In retrospect, that student was a bit of a free spirit and just friendly to everyone. If I had to guess, I think she just wanted to hang out in a platonic manner—especially since I have not had any other invitations to dates since then from anyone other than my wife.

REVIEW OF DEFINITIONS AND NEW TERMINOLOGY

In Chapter 2, we defined *implicit biases* as unconscious preferences or stereotypes that grow either from a lack of interaction with a group or from the life sum of interactions with that group.[3,4] These *stereotypes* are generalizations that do not consider the unique individuals within that demographic. *Explicit biases* are similar except that they are at the conscious level, and the person is aware of their stereotypes, beliefs, and partialities.

In Chapter 3, we also discussed that many people's definitions of racism center around individual negative explicit biases—known as *prejudices*—against a racial or ethnic group, often accompanied by hatred of that group or a belief that the group is inherently inferior.[5] We countered this definition of racism at the individual level with a definition of *systemic racism*, defined by Dr. Camara Jones as "a system of structuring opportunity and assigning value based on the social interpretation of how one looks."[6] Systemic racism does not require any specific malicious intent, and we discussed that a focus on individual racism can sometimes distract from larger and more powerful system issues.

A focus on systemic inequities, with the goal of using system change to eliminate disparities and overcome individual behavior, is the paradigm that we will use for the remainder of this book. Along those same lines, we will center the bulk of this chapter's discussions of sexism around *systemic sexism*. Using the same wording for systemic racism, sexism is a system of structuring opportunity based on the social assignment of gender. The distinctions between sex, gender, gender identity, and gender expression will be examined further in the next chapter. For now, this chapter considers sexism to denote systemic bias against people who self-identify as women as well as against people who are typically perceived by society to be female.

References to women (or girls if below age eighteen) in this chapter are inclusive of everyone within this characterization—even non-binary individuals—since most of the available data on sexism is collected in this binary format. Also, the impacts of systemic bias in society are often related to perception, or the way that the average person sees you. This is similar to the example from Chapter 1, where dark-skinned people from the Dominican Republic are often referred to as Black in the United States, even if they do not identify as such.

In our discussion of bias and racism so far, I have asserted that intent does not matter; both unconscious and explicit biases cause harm to patients, and systemic inequities worsen the morbidity and mortality of people whether or not the systems are intentionally set up to do so. On an individual level, we have explained how so-called positive stereotypes can still be harmful, even if they center around traits and characteristics that are generally viewed as favorable according to societal standards. A closely related concept in discussing sexism in today's culture is one of hostility versus benevolence.

Hostile sexism is the view that most people think about when hearing the word sexism, wherein a person dislikes women or has a misogynistic and hateful view of them.[7] This view is often accompanied by the idea that women are a threat to men or that they are taking opportunities such as jobs away from them. This is in contrast to *benevolent sexism*, whereby women are viewed as needing protection. This type of sexism is often based on the idea of chivalry and being a gentleman, and it is more likely to be viewed favorably by both women and men.

The reason why this seemingly benevolent view of women can be problematic is because it can be strongly associated with stereotypes of women that do not view them in positions of leadership or in high-earning careers. It does not consider the heterogeneity of women's preferences in how they want to be treated. In settings of healthcare, benevolent sexism can also be linked to a lack of trust that women can reliably make their own sound medical decisions.

ORIGINS OF SEXISM

In many of my didactic sessions and trainings, I have repeatedly declared that a plethora of our implicit biases begin during childhood. One of my colleagues who had heard me mention this several times pointed out a supporting example that they had received from a source that they could not remember. They showed me a photograph of the September 2016 issue of *Girls' Life* magazine side-by-side with the same month's issue of *Boys' Life* magazine (Image 10). As you can see, the girls' magazine focuses on fashion, hair styles, dating and relationships, while the boys' version highlights STEM careers, service, and scholarship.

At the end of Chapter 2, I shared a training exercise that I perform which regularly demonstrates my audience's automatic and unconscious association between male gender and wealth. Even when cloaked in benevolence, images that consistently connect boys and men with intelligence, while women and girls are associated as objects of beauty, begin the process of societal programming of gender roles.

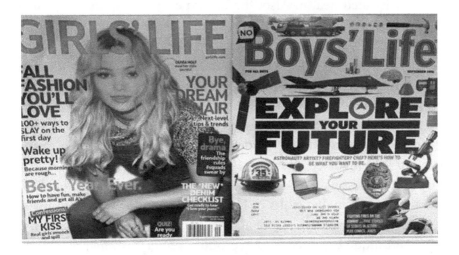

SYSTEMIC SEXISM IN HEALTHCARE

An initial look at the CDC Health Disparities and Inequalities Report paints a picture of women as being clearly healthier than men.[8] They have better outcomes for several metrics, including:

- Longer life expectancy
- Lower suicide and homicide rates
- Lower colon cancer death rates and incidence rates
- Lower death rates from coronary artery disease
- Lower rates of periodontitis
- Better hypertension control.

However, as we discussed in Chapter 1, gender health disparities exist for several measures of morbidity, even as women tend to have better mortality outcomes. In other words, women live longer but they do not always live better. We learned that women have higher rates of certain behavioral health problems such as depression and anxiety, and they are more likely to suffer from domestic abuse. According to the CDC, women often have a lower health-related quality of life, including more physically unhealthy days and more days of "fair" or "poor" self-rated health. Also, the life expectancy gap between men and women has narrowed in recent years because of an increase in deaths linked to both legal and illegal drugs.

In Chapter 2, we explored several instances in which women receive unequal treatment within the healthcare system, including fewer referrals for cardiac catheterization or knee replacement even when presenting with clinical findings similar to men. There are other situations where women tend to receive unequal treatment compared to their male counterparts. For women living with HIV infection, they are less likely to be prescribed antiretroviral therapy (ART), which unsurprisingly results in lower rates of suppressed viral loads in HIV-positive women. There are also clinical disparities associated with the unique experience of reproductive-aged women who have the ability to conceive.

Chapter 3 described how maternal mortality in the United States is worse than in most industrially developed countries around the world. Even before women become pregnant, our fragmented healthcare system does a poor job of providing reliable access to contraception for some women. Data from the CDC's health disparities report,[8] the Committee on Community-Based Solutions to Promote Health Equity in the United States (see Chapter 1),[9] and a supplement on health disparities in women from the journal *Clinical Medicine Insights: Women's Health*[10] demonstrated significant inequities in the following areas:

- Barriers in cancer research
- Reproductive decisions among women living with HIV
- Women living in rural areas
- Lower socioeconomic status women
- Psychosocial and emotional influences on health disparities.

This list of inequities demonstrates a recurring theme that was explored in detail in the Preface and Chapter 1 but has also appeared in each chapter so far. The intersectional nature of human beings is the reason that the chapters in this book do not occur in a uniform or solitary fashion in real life. The experience of a woman living in a rural area or women of low socioeconomic status will be shaped by their gender, their geography, and their financial position, and these confluences of variables come together to affect different people in different ways. Some of these variables, however, seem to have a larger contribution to the largest health inequities.

HIV status has already been mentioned above but, in addition to unequal access to ART, women living with HIV infection often receive discouragement and discrimination when expressing the desire to have children—even when they have undetectable viral loads and carry almost no risk of vertical transmission.

Race is also a unique variable that seems to permeate all aspects of society. In the *Clinical Medicine Insights: Women's Health* journal supplement referred to above, a group of authors asserted:

> *"It should also be noted that the content of this issue is largely rooted in racial/ethnic health disparities. As this was not an intentional focus of the supplement, we feel this may speak to the fact that this area is of high relevance and/or interest to many health investigators due to its public health relevance."*

Noted feminist scholar Kimberlé Crenshaw echoes the sentiment of the strong contribution of race to women's health disparities. Using her theoretical framework of *intersectionality*, Crenshaw details how multiple aspects of a person's social context combine ("intersect") to shape their experience.[11] Any component of a person's identity has the potential to create opportunities for advantage or privilege in some environments, while these characteristics can lead to disadvantage and discrimination in other settings. The components of the intersectionality framework include the following demographic categories:

- Sex
- Sexual orientation
- Gender/gender identity
- Race/ethnicity
- Religion
- Country of origin
- Physical appearance
- Disability status
- Income/socioeconomic status

Crenshaw illustrates the pitfalls of treating the components of this framework as "mutually exclusive categories of experience and analysis." Placing these components in silos and analyzing them separately could lead to evaluations of women's experiences that do not include Black women, and to an analysis of the Black population that does not include Black women. The result would be that the unique challenges that African American women face in society would be made invisible, which we already see as Black women are underrepresented in cancer research and other medical studies. Critiques of these analyses might be met with defensive responses that the large number of women and racial minorities proves that they are not exclusionary despite the underrepresentation of Black women. This theme is exemplified by a book title that Crenshaw has alluded to frequently—*All the Women Are White, All the Blacks Are Men, But Some of Us Are Brave.*

COMBATING SEXISM IN HEALTHCARE

The framework introduced in Chapter 3 can also be used as a starting place for addressing systemic sexism in healthcare. This includes measuring institutional bias—in this case, identifying the inequities that exist for women within your patient population or healthcare organization. Individual departments should identify known areas of inequity that are pervasive in their associated specialties or in the diseases and health conditions that they manage most frequently. An example of this would be for emergency departments to evaluate for problems with human trafficking in their patient population. Although people of any sex or gender can become victims of trafficking, cisgender and transgender girls and women are more likely to be targets.

Human trafficking—which includes both sex trafficking and labor trafficking—often go unrecognized despite the fact that an average of five out of every six victims see a health professional during the time that they are in bondage.[12] Nearly two-thirds of trafficking victims specifically visit an emergency department (ED) during captivity, and this is often the first point of contact with the healthcare system for this socially isolated population. ED physicians, advanced practice providers, nurses, and clerical staff all have a responsibility to identify and support potential victims. (For anyone who questions this responsibility, please refer them to the final section of Chapter 1.) We have discussed the use of evidence-based institutional paradigms from organizations such as the AAP and AAMC to combat systemic bias.

In the case of human trafficking, the HEAL Trafficking and Hope for Justice's Protocol Toolkit can be used to implement institutional protocols that will help to overcome individual provider biases and blind spots. We saw how standardized procedures helped to decrease maternal mortality in California; human trafficking protocols create the possibility of intervening appropriately despite the time constraints and distractions of the ED.

For academic health centers and departments of CME, early instruction should include training about the health inequities that women commonly face. For example, when discussing intrapartum obstetrics, the dismal maternal mortality rate in our country should be highlighted along with systemic changes that have been demonstrated to reduce this disparity. A CME event on the use of ART for HIV infection is an ideal time to discuss that women are less likely to receive this life-saving intervention. Using earlier examples from Chapter 2, medical student didactic sessions on the indications for joint replacement in severe knee osteoarthritis should highlight the fact that women are less likely to receive this intervention even when presenting with the same objective findings as men. Hospital quality improvement reviews of cardiac catheterization outcomes should evaluate the distribution of performed procedures by gender to be sure that women are not failing to be offered this diagnostic and treatment method equitably.

While searching for and measuring institutional bias against women, educating on health inequities that affect women, and initiating protocols that can overcome individual biases against women, we must also be sure that the women who work in healthcare are being treated in a just manner. My bungle of the month mentioned my overblown apprehension of being falsely accused of inappropriate interactions with women, but it did not present the perspective of women having to deal with sexual harassment in the workplace.

A survey by the American College of Radiology demonstrated that almost 25 percent of women experienced sexual harassment at work, compared to only 4 percent of men.[13] The Society of Interventional Radiology showed an even more concerning systemic problem with 21 percent of women experiencing sexual harassment during training and a staggering 47 percent dealing with it in practice. We tend to think of students, residents, and fellows as being more vulnerable because of hierarchies and power differentials, but this study shows the opposite; harassment increased after women were finished with their training.

Complicating the matter is the fact that women often feel powerless when bullied or harassed at work. In a summary of these surveys, Dr. Braileanu et alia recounted that only 20–29 percent of victims report harassment in the workplace, and they described several factors that contribute to this hesitancy to report abusers.[13] These reasons include concerns about confidentiality, fear that they will face retaliation, worry that their career or reputation will be damaged, and doubt that they will be taken seriously or that anything will be done to address their troubles. Women also sometimes downplay the seriousness of harassment and mistreatment, especially when the episodes are not sexual in nature.

In addition to facing high rates of harassment at work, women physicians are not compensated equally to men even when performing the same work. A study of women physicians in academic medical centers showed that their mean salary was $51,315 less than that of men physicians.[14] In debates about the gender pay gap, I often hear the argument that women are paid less than men because they work fewer hours, choose careers with lower salaries, or take advantage of part-time opportunities so that they can have children and spend more time with their kids. I have also heard the anecdotal argument that women are less aggressive in salary negotiation and pursuing promotion.

However, even after adjusting for specialty, hours worked, faculty rank, location, and other confounders, women still make $19,878 less than similarly matched male physicians. A survey of 80,000 physicians, which was published in the journal *Health Affairs*, revealed that women make approximately 25 percent less than men, which equates to a $2 million shortfall over a forty-year career.[15] It turns out that women are simply offered lower salaries and less money than male physicians.

Think back to our discussions on implicit bias and the origins of the female stereotype. The way to combat these problems is to create a system that overcomes individual behavior. This could include institutional policies that perform the same type of analysis that is described in the studies above. For example, organizations can perform annual audits of their salaries by gender and correct any pay gaps or wage disparities. Many institutions have rules that actually punish employees for sharing their salary information with other people in the organization, which leads to a lack of transparency about salaries and an inability for women to know when they are being underpaid. Whenever systems are biased, and you add in the danger of the omnipresent implicit biases that we have, it is a recipe for disaster.

I briefly mentioned promotion and its relation to career advancement in academic medical centers, residency programs, and medical schools. These opportunities are often bolstered or enhanced by awards for teaching, service, and clinical excellence. You can probably guess where this is headed, but women physicians are underrepresented among award recipients despite having similar or better academic records throughout their training. (In other words, the gender discrepancy in awards is not explained by one group being smarter than the other.)

Dr. Julie Silver studied awards from the Association of Academic Physiatrists over the preceding four years, and no awards were given to any women.[16] No women received awards in 50 percent of the award categories over the previous decade, and no woman had won the outstanding fellow/resident award since its inception seven years earlier. In case you are rationalizing this by wondering if there are just fewer women represented in this discipline, the AAMC reported that 41 percent of full-time academic physiatrists are currently reported as female.[17] Similarly, women are relatively well-represented in the field of neurology, as the proportion of women neurologists increased from 18 percent to 31.5 percent during a recent study period. However, only between 0 to 18 percent of award recipients from various categories of the American Academy of Neurologists were women.[18] Finally, women were not represented in any of the lifetime achievement awards for twenty-four of the previous twenty-eight years (85.7 percent).

Within a group, experiences vary significantly between individual members, and the experiences of women are particularly diverse given that they are the largest of the target groups discussed in this book, making up more than half of the population. That can make it feel overwhelming to discuss topics like sexism in medicine, as the subject matter could easily take up an entire book on its own. I recommend that after reading this book the first time, any future references to it should consider how all of the chapters might come together to shape the experiences of the people we care for or interact with within the community.

When addressing women's health disparities, think about women who also identify with all of the other chapters in this book. For example, think about the shared experiences of racial and ethnic minority women, women living with disabilities, women living in rural communities, sexual and gender minority women, or women who are also religious minorities. Also, continue to remember a common theme of this book that, even within these subgroups, there is guaranteed to be significant heterogeneity despite many frequently shared outcomes and experiences.

KNOWLEDGE, ATTITUDES, AND SKILLS

Knowledge

- As with systemic racism, the healthcare system—similar to the rest of the world—can be structurally sexist so that women have fewer opportunities or are assigned lower value based on their gender.

- Systemic sexism > Individual sexism – again paralleling racism, structural and systemic sexism might not invoke as much conscious emotional hurt as individual acts of hostile sexism, but they can still be more damaging on a global scale.

- The concept of intersectionality is even more important in women's health disparities, with inequities that are more glaring when viewing sex and gender together along with race, geographic location, and socioeconomic status.

Attitudes

- The same systemic approach to racism and other health disparities should be used in eradicating systemic sexism, including a deliberate effort to look for and measure institutional bias.

- Benevolent sexism, which is often steeped in good intentions and the concept of chivalry, is frequently harmful by generalizing the intentions of the group and creating implicit and explicit stereotypes of gender roles.

- Tracking of outcomes for women and patients in your organization should consider intersectionality, as women may have different experiences based on their gender in combination with other demographic aspects.

Skills

- Utilize the same paradigms discussed previously to eliminate systemic biases. Measure institutional sexism and create departmental-specific priorities for addressing health inequities.

- While focusing on the system, continue to hold members of your professional community responsible for addressing their individual biases through perpetual self-reflection in addition to team-based events. This includes the previously discussed bias-reducing strategies of individuating, perspective-taking, and exploring how biases contribute to health disparities in your field.

- Integrate women's health equity while addressing disparities for *every other target group*. For example, if you are exploring disability-related inequities, be sure to explore the unique experience of disabled women.

- Be intentional in seeking out women for leadership positions.

- Pay women the same thing that you pay men.

- Have a zero-tolerance policy for tolerating sexual harassment and proactively tell women in your organization about this expectation.

HOW TO TEACH ABOUT SEXISM IN MEDICINE

Although several of our solutions focus on systemic change, we should remember the contributions that our individual behaviors and beliefs have in supporting and preserving unjust systems. Prior to your session on sexism in medicine, encourage your participants to visit the website https://implicit.harvard.edu/implicit/takeatest.html and take the Gender-Career Implicit Association Test (IAT). Ask for volunteers to share their results but be willing to share yours first to help "break the ice." As described at the beginning of Chapter 2, making yourself vulnerable and sharing this type of information about yourself with your participants can help to decrease anxiety, open up dialogue, and make the session less intimidating. For example, upon taking the

Gender-Career IAT, I received the result, "Your data suggest a strong automatic association for Male with Career and Female with Family." I often joke around that we are doing this session so that everyone does not end up like me.

I have used the example from the end of Chapter 2—the implicit bias exercise about the "greedy billionaire"—to teach about implicit biases toward women. This works very well when discussing fair hiring practices or salary negotiation policies for healthcare organizations. It also works well when discussing the selection process for members of the admissions committees and selection committees of people involved in undergraduate and graduate medical education. This exercise is also complemented nicely with a discussion of the "Origins of Sexism," as described earlier in this chapter with the example of the boys' and girls' magazine covers.

This chapter is heavily data-driven, so I tend to use more slide shows and presentations for this material. However, instead of just lecturing on the data, it is more engaging to utilize active learning and explore what your participants' opinions are of the issues as you describe the evidence. I have used audience response systems frequently for this section and for Chapter 6 so that the audience can answer anonymously and avoid potential embarrassment. If your organization does not own an audience response system with handheld remotes, there are a number of free online programs you can use whereby participants text their answers through their cell phones. Here is one example of a question that I have utilized in the past to discuss the gender pay gap for physicians:

- Studies of women physicians in academic medical centers show that they make (on average) $19,878 less (almost $20,000 less!) than male physicians. What is the most likely reason for this?

  A) They are more likely to work part-time after having children.

  B) They are simply offered lower salaries/less money than male physicians.

C) They tend to be less aggressive with pursuing promotion/tenure so that they can focus on family.

D) Studies that show this are skewed/biased and don't consider work hours, geographic location, faculty rank, etc.

After reading this chapter, you know that the answer is "B." I have used both humor and audience participation to keep everyone engaged. For example, I often ask the women in the audience to raise their hands if they would like to make $20,000 less than the men sitting next to them for doing the same job. If you know the audience participants personally and have established trust with them, it is sometimes fun to call one of the men by name (e.g., "To the women and non-men in the group, who doesn't mind making $20,000 less than Bonzo for doing the same job? Really? No one? Are you sure?").

CHAPTER 6

SEXUAL AND GENDER MINORITES (LGBTQ+ HEALTH DISPARITIES)

In 2016, I was awarded the first year of a grant from Frontlines of Communities in the US (FOCUS). As the principal investigator (PI), I was part of a team that received more than $1 million in funding over four years to implement universal, opt-out testing for HIV and Hepatitis C virus (HCV) infection in non-traditional sites. We began testing patients in the ED, using age-based guidelines from the CDC and US Preventive Services Task Force (USPSTF), even if the patients were coming in for a chief complaint that did not raise suspicion for an infectious disease. Georgia has consistently had the highest incidence rate of new HIV infection among all states in the country for the past few years (Image 11),[1] so I took great pride in being able to screen an average of 15,000 people per year in my home state.

I was also motivated by a disturbing analysis from the CDC that same year (2016) that reported a one in two lifetime risk of HIV among Black men who have sex with men (MSM) and a one in four lifetime risk among Latino MSM.[2] Patients who tested positive for HIV were rapidly linked to care by our interdisciplinary team, and our public health workers also educated patients who tested negative but had multiple risk factors. We would often recommend pre-exposure prophylaxis (PrEP) as one method of reducing the risk of acquiring HIV infection.

PrEP is a plan of care that includes the use of daily oral antiretroviral medication—traditionally a combination of tenofovir and emtricitabine—to reduce the risk of acquiring HIV infection in HIV-negative individuals.[3] In a landmark study of MSM published in the *New*

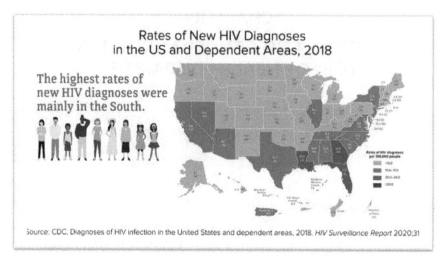

Rates of New HIV Diagnoses
in the US and Dependent Areas, 2018

The highest rates of
new HIV diagnoses were
mainly in the South.

Source: CDC. Diagnoses of HIV infection in the United States and dependent areas, 2018. *HIV Surveillance Report* 2020;31

England Journal of Medicine in 2010, the use of PrEP decreased the incidence of HIV infection by 44 percent.[4] Our grant team became frustrated after receiving call backs from several patients and clients who asked their health care providers for PrEP only to find out it was not available. Using the CDC PrEP locator (https://npin.cdc.gov/preplocator), I discovered that the closest advertised PrEP provider was more than an hour away from our hospital's zip code.

Although I would frequently forget to discuss the option of PrEP with my patients, I would prescribe it for patients who asked about it; I assumed that was the case with most of my colleagues. To my surprise, almost every local physician that I asked did not provide PrEP for their patients for various reasons: they had not been trained on how to do it, they did not feel comfortable prescribing antiretroviral medications because of fear of side effects, they just did not think about it, or they did not think that their patient population was high risk in the state with the highest incidence rate of HIV!

I made it my mission to increase the provision of PrEP in the community, so I arranged PrEP training for my clinic, a federally qualified health center (FQHC), and began to offer the service more frequently. I also provided training for three of the residency clinics—family medicine, internal medicine, and obstetrics and gynecology (OB/GYN)—at the institution where I am on faculty. Our family medicine residency clinic and both of our community's FQHCs are listed on two different PrEP locators now (the CDC locator and Emory University's locator [https://preplocator.org]), along with the county health department and other local offices who started providing PrEP independent of our efforts. The excitement from this progress lured me right into my bungle of the month.

I was seeing a young adult African American man for an annual physical, and he was in good health and living a healthy lifestyle. He mentioned his brand-new boyfriend in passing, so my mind went towards the aforementioned one in two lifetime risk of HIV in Black MSM in the United States. I began to discuss the high incidence of HIV in our state and informed him about the risks and benefits of PrEP. I described the process of monitoring renal function, screening for sexually transmitted infections (STIs), and scheduling outpatient visits every three months for medication prescriptions.

He patiently listened to my five-minute spiel then thanked me for sharing the information with him. He said that he had never heard of PrEP and was amazed that there was a pill that could prevent HIV. He then replied, "Wow. If I ever decide to become sexually active, do I just call you, or would I need to schedule a follow-up appointment?" (Huh?!) I responded back, "So you're not sexually active right now?" to which he informed me, "No, I'm a virgin. I was planning on waiting until I get married to have sex, but I know that sometimes people plan on that, and it doesn't happen." I told him that he could schedule a follow-up if he ever needed it, and he left the encounter as if nothing had happened.

I am not sure if he was just trying to be nice or if he was oblivious to the fact that my implicit bias heard "Black. Male. Gay. Georgia" and immediately stereotyped him as being at risk for HIV. The clinic nurse that I always work with does a detailed sexual history during the intake for all patients, and it was clear as day on his chart that he had never had sex before. I just looked right over it when I saw that he was attracted to men, and I did not bother to ask when he mentioned the new boyfriend.

I jumped to the need for PrEP, but likely missed an opportunity to discuss PrEP with several heterosexual patients that day; several studies have demonstrated the benefits of PrEP for high-risk heterosexual women and for all populations.[5,6] A gay couple comprised of two monogamous HIV-negative men have no risk compared to a straight woman who has condomless sex with men.

Our unconscious biases cause us to stereotype certain patients as being high risk, while not recognizing that people in other demographic groups are actually more at risk. The silver lining is that this implicit bias was revealed to my conscious mind, so I now always double check sexual histories before launching into any future diatribes about PrEP.

DEFINITIONS AND AFFIRMING TERMINOLOGY

Several years ago, I remember the acronym LGBT—lesbian, gay, bisexual, and transgender—being used to refer to people who did not identify as heterosexual. Since then, this acronym has evolved into LGBTQIAP, or LGBTQ+ for short. By the time of publication of this book, it may have changed yet again. Below are a few brief descriptions of how the individual components of the acronym are typically used. Keep in mind a common theme from this book about the heterogeneity of most groups and be aware that everyone might not define these terms the same way.

- Lesbian – women who are sexually or romantically attracted to other women.

- Gay – a term previously used to encompass all people sexually attracted to the same gender, but now predominantly used for men who are sexually or romantically attracted to other men (see below for more details on romantic versus sexual attraction). Some MSM do not identify as gay if they do not experience romantic attraction to men.

- Bisexual – people who are sexually attracted to men and women. They may be romantically attracted to only men, only women, or both. Some people use this term to specify people whose romantic and sexual partners are cisgender, which could differentiate them from pansexual individuals.

- Transgender – people whose gender identity does not match their sex assigned at birth.

- Queer – similar to the historical use of the term gay, queer may be used as an umbrella term for non-heterosexual people, but it typically also includes non-cisgender people. The majority of people who identify as queer are cisgender women and non-binary people who do not conform to male or female identity. In the past, queer was used as a pejorative term.

  - GQNB – emerging term for genderqueer/non-binary individuals who identify as both masculine and feminine.

- Questioning – people who do not fit into a specific group but are not sure if they conform to traditional cisgender/heterosexual ("cis-het") categorizations.

- Intersex – people born without fitting all the typical characteristics of any specific sex, especially people who have ambiguous genitalia or the presence of male and female genitalia. The use of the term "hermaphrodite" to describe these individuals is now considered outdated and offensive.

- Asexual/Aromantic – either not attracted to anyone sexually (asexual) or not attracted to people romantically (aromantic or "aro").

  - Allied – sometimes the "A" is used to also refer to people who self-identify as an ally to the LGBTQ+ community, although some people do not endorse this as allies do not experience the same societal challenges as other groups described above.

- Pansexual – sexually and/or romantically attracted to people of any sex or gender.

The Genderbread Person (Image 12) and the Gender Unicorn (Image 13) from the Safe Zone Training Project illustrate the differences between sexual and romantic attraction. They also introduce additional terminology beyond LGBTQ+ (described below) that is required for understanding several concepts that are important in the health equity discussions in this chapter.

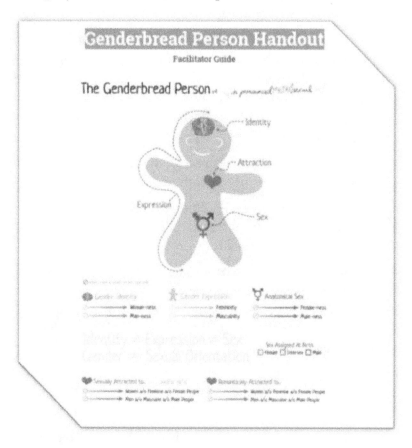

- Gender – assigned as male or female based on a set of physical and psychological characteristics, social behaviors, and traits that are considered masculine or feminine, respectively, by societal standards.

- Gender identity – the gender that a person identifies as, regardless of how they are perceived by others. If this matches their sex assigned at birth, then they are referred to as *cisgender*.

- Gender expression – focuses on how a person appears based on social behaviors associated with particular genders; this includes social behaviors, manner of dress, and speech patterns. People who do not fit into either category or who are "gender-fluid" are often referred to as *androgynous*.

- Sex – the binary gender, either male or female, that is assigned at birth. This is typically based on anatomical sex and external genitalia, as opposed to being defined genetically or based on chromosomal analysis.

- Sexual orientation – gender that people are sexually attracted to.

A review article written by Brittany Bass and Hassan Nagy is available online at StatPearls, and it defines the terms above in detail along with several other terms that I did not include.[7]

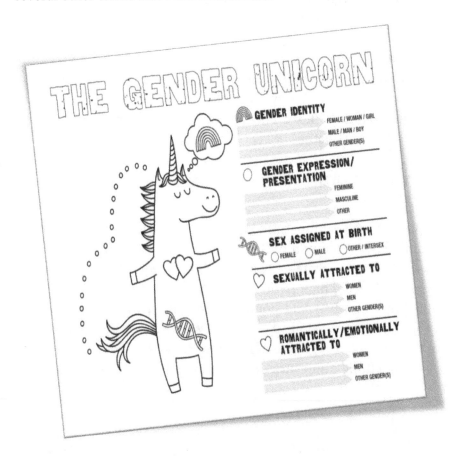

Some people who might appear to fit into one of the categories of the LGBTQ+ acronym may not identify as such,[8] which is why the National Institutes of Health (NIH) and others use more general categories to identify individuals with unique health needs based on their gender, sexual orientation, or other characteristics.[9,10] The term sexual and gender minorities (SGM) is defined by the NIH as follows:

> *"SGM populations include, but are not limited to, individuals who identify as lesbian, gay, transgender, two-spirit, queer, and/ or intersex. Individuals with same-sex or gender attractions or behaviors and those with a difference in sex development are also included. These populations also encompass those who do not self-identify with one of these terms but whose sexual orientation, gender identity or expression, or reproductive development is characterized by non-binary constructs of sexual orientation, gender, and/or sex."*

This book at times uses the acronym LGBTQ+ synonymously with SGM, with the "+" symbol recognizing not only individuals in the "IAP" portion of the acronym but also anyone included in the NIH definition who does not identify with the other components of the LGBTQIAP abbreviation.

HEALTH INEQUITIES AMONG SEXUAL AND GENDER MINORITIES

Chapter 1 briefly summarized the health disparities report from the Committee on Community-Based Solutions to Promote Health Equity in the United States.[11] Notable LGBTQ+ health disparities described included a high frequency of markers of low socioeconomic status—more poverty and homelessness—as well as adverse behavioral health outcomes linked to stigma. We have already discussed the disproportionately high rate of HIV among MSM—especially among racial and ethnic minorities—but sexual and gender minorities also have higher rates of other sexually transmitted infections (STIs) compared to other people in the population.

According to systematic reviews, LGBTQ+ youth and adolescents are also at higher risk of sexual assault, bullying, family rejection, and chemical dependency.[12] Up to 40 percent of sexual minority youth experience homelessness, and two-thirds do not discuss their sexual orientation with their health care providers. The 2019 Behavioral Risk Factor Surveillance System survey demonstrated that health inequities persist into late adulthood, with studies of LGBTQ+ adults aged fifty years and older revealing poor access to preventive medical care, higher prevalence of disabilities, and the same high rates of poor physical and mental health seen in younger SGM people.[13]

There are some glaring health inequities specific to certain subgroups within the LGBTQ+ community, such as disparities in cervical cancer screening among lesbian women and transgender men (assigned female sex at birth). Most cases of cervical cancer are caused by human papillomavirus (HPV), which is traditionally thought of as being spread through sexual contact involving male and female genitalia. As a result, many health care providers incorrectly believe that lesbian women or people who do not have sex with men do not need to be screened via cervical cytology (PAP smears) and HPV testing. This does not consider the fact that many lesbian women have had sex with men in their lifetimes or that some sexual practices between lesbian women can spread HPV.

The result is that screening rates for cervical cancer among women who have sex with women are barely half of the rates for heterosexual women despite the fact that almost one-third of lesbian women test positive for HPV in some studies. This is the reason that the USPSTF recommends cervical cancer screening for everyone who has a cervix and is between the ages of 21 and 65.[14]

I have met several lesbian patients who either believed that they did not need to be screened or had been told by a physician that they did not need to receive PAP smears. This is consistent with qualitative studies of lesbian women in the United States and in other countries, which also outline mistrust of health care providers and fear of pain with speculum exams as additional barriers to screening.[15-17] Transgender men often have the same experiences, and this is likely compounded if they have a masculine gender expression.[18] The same situation occurs among transgender and transmasculine men when it comes to contraception, as some patients receiving testosterone therapy mistakenly believe—or are told by their provider—that they cannot become pregnant, or they believe that testosterone is a form of birth control.[19] They also frequently assume that amenorrhea is a sign of infertility.

In an effort to provide gender-affirming care, physicians can sometimes forget about the reproductive organs still present in their patients' bodies. For example, they may almost forget that a transgender man still has a uterus and can become pregnant, or that a transgender woman still has a prostate gland that can develop cancer.

I was once finishing up a patient encounter with a transgender man when his partner nervously whispered something to him. I could tell something was bothering them, so I asked if there was something else they wanted to discuss. My patient mentioned that he was interested in a copper intrauterine device (IUD) for birth control. Similar to my bungle of the month from earlier in this chapter, I had reviewed my patient's sexual history on that day but did not pay as close attention to it as I should have. I saw that my patient was a transgender man who identified as gay, which led to an assumption that he was not having receptive vaginal intercourse. It turned out that he was, and they had concerns about the possibility of pregnancy.

I had heard some transgender patients express disdain for the reproductive organs that they were born with, so I think I used that to stereotype all of my transmasculine patients as not deriving pleasure from sexual activity involving their vaginas. Fortunately, my patient's partner spoke up as an advocate, and I was able to place his IUD on that same day. Since then, I have tried to be even more cognizant of the heterogeneity of the reproductive health needs of sexual and gender minority populations.

These examples highlight the need for culturally competent clinicians who will know what questions to ask, and whose patients will trust them enough to remind them if they forget to ask these questions. Many of the disparities discussed so far are rooted in mistrust of health care providers and stigma associated with people's sexuality and gender identity. There is also a need for healthcare and educational systems that create safety nets for the individual blind spots of biased individuals.

Chapter 8 will discuss *cultural competence* in depth; for now, think of it in the way that it is defined by Drs. Melanie Tervalon and Jann Murray-Garcia as inquiring about, responding to, and respecting patients' beliefs and desires.[20] Over time, this will result in a better understanding about trends among certain cultural groups, and it will create a competence in how to manage conditions that are prevalent in these populations. In the chapter on cultural competence, we will also discuss the importance of cultural humility which recognizes the differences *within* groups and appreciates the need to treat each person as an individual—a theme that this book has hopefully established so far.

COMBATING SYSTEMIC BIAS AGAINST SEXUAL AND GENDER MINORITIES

By now you can probably predict where the process begins in combating systemic bias against the LGBTQ+ community. As we have said since Chapter 3, the strategic plan to eliminate inequities should be presented in a way that demonstrates how it aligns with the institutional mission and vision of the organization. In line with the themes that have been presented so far, we should promote organizational diversity and encourage sexual and gender minorities to apply for employment and leadership opportunities to ensure that they have a voice.

Given the stigma that these populations consistently face, this requires a proactive statement that people will be accepted and embraced regardless of sexual orientation or gender identity. We should also compensate them when they are asked to give feedback about how to improve processes, as opposed to seeking them out for free advice. Next, it is important to reach an agreement on institutional definitions and standards. Similar to how we discussed coming to a consensus about how we define race and racism, we should agree upon affirming terminology for sexual and gender minorities and agree upon language that is unacceptable.

After setting formal standards for an inclusive environment and defining your purpose through the lens of your organizational mission, the next goal is to address specific disparities by making system changes. Using the contraception example described above, system changes might involve continuing medical education for providers within your organization to learn about family planning for transgender individuals. Chance Krempasky et al. detail the need for research in this area, in addition to education about drug interactions with hormone therapy, so these should be institutional priorities for academic health centers, medical schools, etc.[21]

Many physicians and advanced practice providers that I have met do not feel comfortable treating transgender men and women, and they are often unaware of the existence of guidance from organizations such as the World Professional Association for Transgender Health (WPATH).[22] There has been a significant improvement in evidence-based guidelines on the medical management of sexual and gender minorities, but notable expert Kathleen Bonvicini describes slow progress in cultural competency education.[23] Similar to the "silent curriculum" that Katherine Brooks mentioned in medical schools (see Chapter 3), we have a lot of information about the health inequities facing LGBTQ+ populations without guidance about how to improve the education of the physicians and nurses caring for them.

As with the approach to eliminating other health disparities, this process has to be intentional; healthcare organizations have to go hunting for inequities. They must have a policy or clear stance on the clinical care and treatment of sexual and gender minorities so that there is not inconsistency in providers' willingness to care for them. Individual academic departments should again identify the health inequities that exist within their specialties. There are parallels between this chapter and Chapter 5, in that we must support our employees, faculty, students, and staff who are members of these historically marginalized and excluded groups.

In the previous chapter, we discussed supporting women in our organizations by having zero tolerance for sexual harassment and by eliminating gender-based wage gaps. For the LGBTQ+ members of our work and educational communities, we need reliable and effective ways for them to report concerns anonymously, and for people who do not wish to remain anonymous we must prevent retaliation when complaints are filed. We must also support and assist them when they are mistreated by patients.

In an article in the *New York Times Magazine,* Kwame Appiah mentioned that episodes of patient bias against health care professionals can be "wounding."[24] Although his article focused on race and gender, I have witnessed verbal abuse from patients when a male physician on our inpatient team was deemed to be effeminate by a patient. The AAMC Institutional Diversity Paradigm that we introduced in Chapter 3 included serving diverse populations as one of its goals.[25] Some of the populations we care for have had less exposure to people from various backgrounds, but this is not an excuse to allow homophobic speech to be directed to our team members.

I believe that speech does not have to be violent or profane to be unacceptable, so I have always immediately insisted that patients stop any abusive language. However, I have heard from several of our resident physicians that they do not always receive the benefit of this type of intervention because we are so often taught to prioritize patient satisfaction. As discussed in Chapter 2, the quadruple aim of healthcare should also take into consideration the emotional well-being of the people delivering the medical care.

Our LGBTQ+ medical students also need support, as mistreatment during their undergraduate medical education can have lasting effects into residency and beyond. The Medical Student Cognitive Habits and Growth Evaluation (CHANGE) Study revealed increased risk of depression, anxiety, and poor health for sexual and gender minority medical students.[26] The same factors that create an inclusive hospital and clinic environment are important in creating a positive learning environment. The AAMC published a resource for medical educators that discusses both curricular and institutional climate changes that can improve the care of LGBTQ+ patients and people born with differences of sex development (DSD, often included in the category intersex).[27] They recommend targeting everyone, including students, faculty, and administrators, and using medical education as an inroad to address health disparities.

INCLUSIVE CLINICAL BEHAVIORS

A thorough sexual history for all patients—not just sexual and gender minorities—should evaluate for family planning and contraceptive needs, sexual behavior, and sexually transmitted infection (STI) risk. The FQHC where I have worked for the past few years accomplishes this with a list of questions that are asked of every patient at their outpatient encounters regardless of the reason for their visit. Making these questions standard for every patient decreases the potential for the clinician to allow their implicit bias to either elevate or minimize a patient's risk. It also decreases stigma or patients' hesitancy to answer accurately when they realize that the questions are asked of all patients.

Our front desk documents patients' pronouns in order to confirm their gender identity. During the triage process, the nurses collect three bundles of information, displayed below via screenshots from the CompuGroup Med (CGM) electronic medical record system. *Family Planning Annual Report (FPAR) Data* are required of all organizations that receive grants from Title X for family planning services (see https://fpar.opa.hhs.gov/). The FPAR questionnaire (Image 14) includes the following questions:

- Are you sexually active? {yes/no}
- Are you planning to have a child within the next one year? {yes/no/not sure}

- What is your primary method of birth control? {drop down menu for all available categories, including hormonal, non-hormonal, and natural family planning methods}

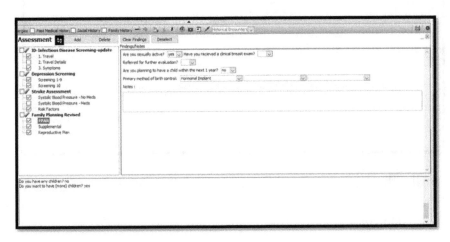

The supplement to the FPAR questionnaire includes the following questions (Image 15):

- How many children do you have?
- How many sexual partners have you had in the past year?
- Do you ever use condoms?
- Date of last unprotected sexual encounter? *(Dr. Quinton Robinson, an infectious disease specialist in Atlanta and one of my classmates from medical school, convinced me to start using the term "condomless" sex instead of unprotected sex, as it has less of an accusatory tone to it and is less stigmatizing. I do not have a reference but just trust me, he told me).*
- Are you concerned about getting pregnant?
- Have you ever had a sexually transmitted disease/infection (STD/STI)?
- Date of last menstrual period?
- Have you ever had sex with a man, a woman, or both?
- Have you ever had vaginal, anal, or oral sex?

111

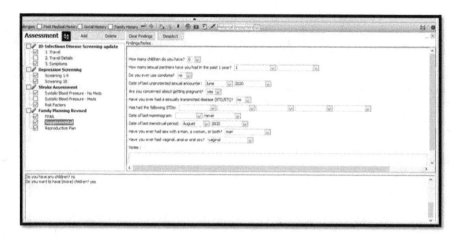

Finally, the Reproductive Plan asks the following questions (Image 16):

- Do you have any children?
- Do you want to have (more) children?
- (If yes) How many (more) children would you like to have?
- When would you like to have more children?

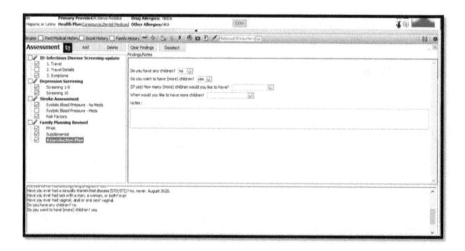

Predetermined questionnaires such as the ones above get around our individual biases that sometimes assume that cisgender heterosexual women all want to have children or that women with masculine gender expressions do not want children. Although they lengthen the triage process, that time is regained by shortening the physician encounter and creating easier transitions into more in-depth questions about sexuality and reproduction.

KNOWLEDGE, ATTITUDES, AND SKILLS

Knowledge

- Our biases can affect the way we care for/work with people. They can also impair the learning environment of medical education and create long-lasting deleterious effects in our LGBTQ+ students and residents.
- Words matter! Not using inclusive language can interfere with rapport-building with our patients and colleagues.
- Instances of bias/mistreatment have an adverse effect on the clinical environment.

Attitudes

- Perpetual self-assessment and reflection is key. People tend to correct their biased behavior once they become aware of it.
- Try not to be offended when you are confronted about biases that you have.
- While being aware of cultural differences and trends, focus on the individual patient!

Skills

- Use the same institutional paradigm discussed in previous chapters to promote health equity for LGBTQ+ populations.
    - Measure institutional bias against sexual and gender minorities.
    - Create institutional standards on acceptable language.
    - Address the system and the individual.

- Spend time with people that are different than you. This is especially true with regard to transgender people, who have some of the worst experiences with stigma in healthcare and adverse behavioral health outcomes.

HOW TO TEACH ABOUT HOMOPHOBIA AND TRANSPHOBIA

Using the same website that we recommended in the last chapter for the Sexism in Medicine discussion, have your participants visit https://implicit.harvard.edu/implicit/takeatest.html and take the Sexuality Implicit Association Test (IAT). Again, I encourage you to lead the way and break down any barriers of fear or shame by sharing your results with the audience. Unfortunately, my IAT results told me, "Your responses suggested a strong automatic preference for straight people over gay people."

In Chapter 5, I offered up to you a self-deprecating joke that this is why we do bias training. If you have done multiple sessions with the same group, you can follow that up with a joke that you might not be invited back if you do not start getting better grades. At the same time, you can reassure anyone else who scored as poorly that, at the time I took the Sexuality IAT, only 18 percent of people score the coveted "little or no automatic preference for straight people compared to gay people."

The Safe Zone Project (https://thesafezoneproject.com) describes itself as a "free, online resource for powerful, effective LGBTQ awareness and ally training workshops." They are an excellent resource for information about terminology and cultural issues to be aware of. They also have several training ideas and illustrations that can assist you in your discussions.

Earlier in this chapter, we referenced the AAMC's resource for medical educators on curricular and institutional climate changes that can improve the care of LGBTQ+ patients and people born with DSD.[27] This document is available for free online and uses multimodal curricular integration blended with competency-based education.

It includes eight clinical scenarios along with suggested discussion points that are appropriate for all stages of learning:

1. Gender nonconformity in prepubertal children

2. Gender dysphoria in an adolescent

3. Iatrogenic trauma in a male born with DSD

4. Possible DSD and gender dysphoria in an adolescent

5. A child with two lesbian mothers and two gay fathers

6. HIV risk behaviors in an adult male

7. A straight man who has sex with men and women

8. A transgender man with a pelvic mass

You may also use the following three cases that I have utilized during my health equity trainings. They are based on real-life scenarios that I have witnessed, although I have changed some details to protect the privacy of the people involved.

CASE #1

You are at a work mixer for your outpatient clinic, having a great time. You are excited that one of the new physicians that you interviewed is here. You introduce her to some of the other staff members. She brought her young daughter with her and mentions that her other kid is home sick. One of the nurses jokes around and says, "So your husband got stuck at home with the kid, huh?" She (the new employee) awkwardly laughs and responds, "Yeah." You remember the new physician telling you that she identifies as lesbian and is married to a woman.

- [Big] deal or no [big] deal? Do you say something to your nursing colleague?

CASE #2

You are a medical receptionist, and your clinic's triage nurse is openly gay. They tell you about an encounter with a patient who comes to the clinic frequently. During the intake questioning, the patient is asked about their sexual orientation using the new screening process that was implemented after reading Dr. Bonzo's book. The patient responds, "I am married to a man...the way it should be. Men are supposed to marry women!" The nurse is hurt by this but tells you, "Don't worry, they're always like that."

- How do you respond as a team member? Would your response change if *you* were the nurse? Physician? Clinic executive or medical director?

CASE #3

You are a medical assistant in a pediatric clinic, but it is public knowledge that you are engaged and will be moving to your fiancé's hometown (out of state). You will be applying for a similar position, and the current medical director of your clinic has been mentoring you to ensure success in this process. You expect to receive a strong reference letter. You repeatedly hear this physician making fun of transgender teens. The most egregious example was when he referred to a transgender adolescent as "it" and "shem" (a derogatory term that mixes the pronouns "she" and "him").

- How do you respond? Be honest, would it change if your mentor personally knew the executives at your desired new place of employment?

DISCUSSION

For the three cases, you can use the following discussion points:
- What language can we agree upon as unacceptable?
- What language is clearly acceptable or preferred?
- Are there any gray areas or questions that we aren't sure about?
- What do we do if we feel like novices in this area?

CHAPTER 7

RELIGIOUS TOLERANCE

As you learned during our discussion of Juan Williams and his fear of people in "Muslim garb" (see end of Chapter 3), for my entire life, I have been around friends and family members who follow the practices of Islam. I have heard my uncle remind one of my cousins that he should not be casually dating, and I have heard young ladies be told that it is not appropriate for them to be alone with non-male family members. As a result, it did not surprise me when I started my clinical years during medical school and found that many Muslim women that we saw requested that there be no men present during their evaluations. This was especially common during gynecological or obstetric evaluations that required genitourinary examinations. I came to expect to be asked to step out whenever I saw a patient wearing a hijab or niqab,⁵ and I was not bothered by the request.

Fast forward to several years out of residency, where I was practicing broad-spectrum family medicine at an academic medical center. This included delivering babies in a five-member group of teaching physicians—later expanded to six—and a lot of time spent on the Labor and Delivery (L&D) unit of our women's hospital. One of our patients was a Muslim woman who came to all of her visits with her husband; they did not mind men physicians but requested to have appointments with women physicians on the days that she would be expected to have a pelvic exam (e.g., during the third trimester, when we perform a rectovaginal swab for group B *Streptococcus*).

Unfortunately, prenatal care is unpredictable, and sometimes a symptom or objective finding during the evaluation will prompt a random genitourinary or speculum exam. This would sometimes create awkward scenarios, such as a request from this Muslim family for one of the men in the group to go find a female physician in the practice to perform a sensitive exam. Most of my colleagues would not mind, but you could sometimes sense frustration if they themselves were running behind in clinic and were asked to help out with something basic like a wet prep (saline wet mount) examination to look for a yeast infection.

At the beginning of the third trimester of this patient's pregnancy, our group had discussions about how to handle her intrapartum care once she came in for delivery. One of the women in our faculty group decided that she would come in to supervise her childbirth, even if she was not on call. My colleague only had one short weekend when she had to be out of town, but that was a couple of weeks before her due date. I joked around that this only meant the patient would now go into labor on that exact weekend, and that I was sure that I would be the one on call. Well of course that actually happened!

The patient came into labor a couple of weeks before her due date, but she was still beyond thirty-seven weeks gestation, so she was considered to be full term. I was on call, my partner was out of town just for that weekend, and the other women in the group were unavailable for various legitimate reasons. On top of that, the senior resident physician and the intern who were on call that night…were both men!

I could not believe it when I received the phone call, and my shock turned into mild emotional distress when I learned that the entire three-member call team that night was male. When I arrived at the hospital, I spoke to the charge nurse, and we developed a plan that was acceptable to the patient and her husband. They paired the patient up with one of our most experienced L&D nurses who would perform the cervical checks to assess the patient's progress during labor.

We made it through the first stage of labor, and the patient was fully dilated and ready to deliver. The resident physicians and I stood behind the curtain in the room to give the patient privacy, while the nurse "pushed" with the patient. This is a common practice for uncomplicated deliveries, and the delivering physician or midwife often comes in when the baby is ready to come. The plan was for us to only come out when the fetal head was "crowning," or starting to come out, but of course that would have been too simple.

The fetal heart rate started to drop to an unsafe range, so the nurse called us from behind the curtain to help out. We performed the appropriate interventions and the fetal heart rate returned to a safe range, but the nurse did not feel comfortable with us stepping out of the room or even back behind the curtain. The husband asked me what was going on, and I started to feel anxiety that a confrontation was coming as I explained the various catheters, electrodes, and monitors that we were utilizing.

The patient eventually delivered, and the baby came out looking vigorous and healthy. The father began to pray and give thanks as the mother gently wept tears of joy. The family did not make eye contact with me from the moment the baby was born, so we finished up and I quietly stepped out of the room to check on some of our admissions in other parts of the hospital.

I received a page—remember pagers from back in the day?—from the L&D nurse and she told me that the patient's husband wanted to debrief about how the delivery went. My previous anxiety returned, and I told her that I was busy with some of our non-obstetric patients but would try to stop back later. A little while later, I received another page and the nurse said that the husband really wanted to talk to me about the delivery. The senior resident on call asked if I wanted him to take care of it, but I figured that it was best for me to handle it and stop procrastinating.

As I walked back to L&D, I began to think about how to handle any anger or disappointment the husband might have, and I was ready to engage in the debate about whether they would have preferred more privacy for his wife versus assurance that his baby was healthy. As I entered the unit, the husband happened to be walking out of the room on the way to get a snack. He saw me in the hallway and began grinning from ear to ear. He quickly walked towards me and hugged me, prayed for blessings upon my family and me, and thanked me for everything. He said that he appreciated us respecting their request for modesty, and also understood that we needed to step in at the end when there was a medical risk. I told him that they were more than welcome, and I carried on with an uneventful evening.

This was not as embarrassing of a bungle as some of my others, because most of the bungle happened within my own brain. There was a good outcome, a happy family, and a healthy baby. I have had hundreds of pregnant patients present with birth plans, and some of them were very frustrated when their childbirth experience did not go according to plan. Add to that a strong religious conviction, and I thought that the "curve balls" during this Muslim family's experience was going to make them very unhappy and unsatisfied.

It turned out that I was much more worried about things than they were, and the in-depth discussions that began during faculty meetings months ago were probably a little overblown. This exemplifies a major theme from this book, which is to be aware of cultural trends, but also to treat each person as an individual. I would like to think that I have displayed cultural competence in the care of my Muslim patients, but experience being around them paradoxically led to unnecessary anxiety and preparation for a debate that never happened.

RELIGIOUS BIAS IN HEALTHCARE

We have discussed a definition of systemic bias that includes the existence of disadvantages among certain target groups based on the way the system is structured. So far this has been described in the context of existing objective inequities in health outcomes. We have spent less time discussing subjective experiential differences in outcomes based on spiritual or religious convictions. For example, a religious minority patient could have the same medical outcomes as other groups, but they could still have a poor experience because they were not allowed to receive their medical care in the context that accommodates the way they practice their religion.

The triple aim of healthcare that we have discussed previously includes the patient experience, and Press Ganey Associates (https://www.pressganey.com) has created an entire industry out of administering patient satisfaction surveys. But we have also discussed the quadruple aim of healthcare that additionally considers the experience of the health care provider. Is there a point where an organization draws the line between giving patients dignity in their medical care and letting them dictate every aspect of their care? How should patient requests and a physician's or nurse's emotional well-being intersect?

In the previous chapter, we discussed an article by Kwame Appiah that debated whether patients should be able to choose their physician based on race and gender.[1] When I was a resident, I went in to see a patient on my outpatient schedule, and an older White man was sitting there with his wife. As soon as I entered the room, he developed a stunned look on his face and immediately said, "I'm sorry, I'm not racist or anything but this isn't going to work. I need a White doctor." I said, "Okay, you can go up to the front desk and reschedule with someone else," and I left the room thankful that I was instantaneously caught back up in clinic after previously running thirty minutes behind.

I told my supervising physician—a White woman—what happened so that she would not wonder where the patient had gone, and she became irate. She charged to the front desk to find and confront the patient even though I told her it was not that big of a deal. The patient had already made it out of the building, so she ended up talking to our practice manager. They sent the patient a certified letter saying that we have a diverse physician group, so he would be better served in another clinic. He was given thirty days to find a new health care provider. I thought it was overkill, but I appreciated the support from my White colleagues.

Every Black physician that I have ever asked has had a similar occurrence to the one described above, but I have not known almost any White physicians who have been told to their face by a patient that they do not want a White doctor. Interestingly, I have heard from front desk staff at various clinics that new patients often call asking if there are any Black physicians. When I have polled my audiences during speaking engagements, they often find no problem with Black patients requesting Black physicians, but they are offended by a White patient saying that they do not want a Black physician.

The rationale for this is often steeped in the history of mistreatment of racial and ethnic minorities in the United States, so people express understanding of a desire for a Black doctor. Similarly, most people understand when a woman asks for a woman physician for their gynecological exam, especially when the patient has a history of being sexually abused. A Muslim patient requesting a male or female provider is often considered another one of these acceptable patient requests, but most of my audiences are not comfortable with a patient saying that they do not want a Muslim provider. This highlights how complex and nuanced discussions are with regard to patient requests for their health care providers.

Some patients have implicit or explicit bias that they do not verbally or openly express, and sometimes requests for new physicians are based on concerns that the patient "just felt uncomfortable" with their doctor. We discussed Mr. Appiah's description that patient bias against, and mistreatment of, physicians can be "wounding," and his article gave several examples. He described a doctor who experienced patients and their families insisting on "having medical providers who are some combination of straight, White, male and/or American born." He questioned if it was ethical to allow patients' "bigotry [to] dictate who treats them," or for organizations to support patient decisions that are "based on bias."

These are discussions that require a significant amount of thought and energy so that a fair and reasonable conclusion is reached. That is why it is critical to proactively develop institutional policies ahead of time rather than waiting to react when one of these uncomfortable situations arises. For example, the Appiah article described White patients who did not want any Black doctors or nurses to touch them or their family members. He rhetorically questioned if accommodating requests like this was a way of creating institutional bias. His conclusion puts the power into the hands of the person being discriminated against, as the staff member might not want to interact with a patient who is openly displaying bias toward them. This might be more important than any concerns about letting the biased patient "win."

Although several examples above describe bias against someone based on race and ethnicity, religious intolerance, racism, and xenophobia are often destructive partners that do their damage concurrently. Bias from patients towards physicians should not be tolerated, and neither should bias from physicians toward their patients. I have never heard of a physician requesting to not see a patient based on their religion or country of origin, but I have heard stories about physicians making insensitive jokes about colleagues based on these factors. One of my past colleagues from the Middle East said that his boss once joked around that he looked like a "terrorist" when he grew his beard out.

Systemic bias creates an environment where my colleague did not feel that they could safely challenge someone above them in the hierarchical structure, and where the system did not preemptively educate employees about avoiding discriminatory language. There has been an increase in Islamophobia across the globe over the past few decades, and this has a negative effect on the mental health and health behaviors (a social determinant of health) of patients and employees.[2] As such, combating discrimination based on religion should be a part of any institutional diversity plan using the same systemic approach discussed in other chapters of this book so far.

In addition to reducing bias against patients based on faith and religion, a culturally competent approach to the health care of religious minorities should also be a part of any organizational action plan. For example, a primary care or endocrinology clinic should be aware of the impact of Ramadan on Muslim patients with diabetes mellitus. Ramadan is the eleventh month of the Islamic calendar, and it is a time when Muslims fast from dawn until sunset, avoiding food, drink, and physical intimacy.

Studies of Muslim diabetic patients during Ramadan have revealed a 7.5-fold increase in hypoglycemia, as well as an increased risk of kidney stones, especially in hot climates.[3,4] Hydrating aggressively in the early morning prior to sunrise is one way of mitigating the kidney stone risk. The risk of hypoglycemia can be minimized by decreasing basal insulin by 25–50 percent and avoiding the use of mealtime insulin during the hours that patients are fasting. Also, if a patient is taking oral diabetes meds that carry a high hypoglycemia risk (e.g., sulfonylureas, meglitinides), they can be transitioned to medications that carry less risk such as metformin or incretin mimetics.

Fasting is generally not recommended for type 1 diabetics, and Islam does exempt individuals from fasting and from the Hajj if they have medical contraindications, if they are frail, or if they are in poor health. In my experience, some patients will not voluntarily excuse themselves from fasting, but they are willing to do so if encouraged by a trusted and culturally competent physician.

The concept of intersectionality that we have discussed repeatedly so far should illuminate the complexity in discussing religious health disparities. For example, there are more than one billion practicing Muslims worldwide, and their experiences within healthcare systems will also be influenced by gender, country of origin, current geographic location, socioeconomic status, race, ethnicity, and numerous other social and demographic factors.

In a systematic review from 2015 involving 171 studies, South Asians and Arabs were the most studied groups with large Muslim populations.[5] The most common nations represented in studies of Muslims were Somalia, Bosnia, and Afghanistan. Overall, the study determined that there was not a clear connection between the Islamic faith and any specific health outcomes. In another study on religion and chronic disease, Nowakowski and Sumerau studied sixteen common chronic diseases and stratified patients by religion—Catholic, Protestant, Jewish, Other, and None.[6] After adjusting for other non-religious demographic factors, there was no significant difference in the prevalence of chronic disease or in other health outcomes.

RELIGIOUS TOLERANCE IN HEALTHCARE

In an article in the *Annals of Internal Medicine*, Paul-Emile and co-authors offer recommendations for medical centers on explicitly addressing patient bias toward health care workers.[7] As with the other paradigms introduced in this book so far, they recommend a systematic approach that includes trusted mechanisms for reporting grievances coupled with support for those who file reports. In keeping with our recommendation to be proactive, the approach should include training on how to confront bias-based patient behavior, both from the standpoint of the target and from the standpoint of bystanders. They also recommend that medical centers generally reject requests for clinician reassignment that are based on explicit bias. According to this approach, requests to switch physicians or other health care providers should only be allowed for "clinically indicated concordance," such as a patient seeking a doctor who speaks their native language.

Patient requests and behaviors that stem from a psychiatric condition (e.g., PTSD) are often permitted and excused, as they are considered to be beyond the patient's complete control. We discussed that sex or gender concordance for sensitive exams involving patients who are survivors of sexual assault are often deemed understandable. So, if a patient requested a female provider because of a past history of sexual assault by a man, few people would challenge that request. However, these types of requests can be distressing to the health care team or the system if they are correlated with religion, race, or ethnicity.

Using the same example, if a woman was assaulted by a specific member of a racial group and said that they did not want to see any provider of that same race, there is considerable debate about whether or not this is acceptable. This also raises the question of whether we have the right or responsibility to ask "Why?" when a patient requests a new provider. In general, policies should ultimately recognize a patient's past experiences, including discrimination, in any decision-making processes, while also maintaining patient privacy and autonomy. At the same time, they should not allow language or verbal expressions that are openly biased or prejudiced.

When patients are openly discriminatory towards members of the medical team, the protection of staff must be done in a way that does not violate federal law. The Emergency Medical Treatment and Labor Act (EMTALA) requires facilities to provide stabilizing care to everyone experiencing a medical emergency. Title VII of the Civil Rights Act of 1964 prohibits discrimination based on race, sex, religion, or national origin, so medical facilities must be sure that the denial of patient's requests are not seen as violating an individual's right to practice their religion.

The Mayo Clinic developed a five-step policy for responding to bias incidents (Image 17) that considers the potentially competing interests of the patient, the members of the health care team, the healthcare organization as an entity, and the mission of the healthcare organization.[8] This policy addresses two main situations: (1) patient requests for specific characteristics of care team (race, *religion*, ethnicity, gender identity, sexual orientation), or (2) behavior of a discriminatory, harassing, or demeaning manner towards staff. Their training involves use of the "SAFER" mnemonic as a means of developing a standardized approach to addressing patient behavior. The components of the five-step "SAFER" model are as follows:

- S   Step in when you see a problem
- A   Address the inappropriate behavior
- F   Focus on institutional values
- E   Explain policy/expectations
- R   Report the incident to your supervisor (document!)

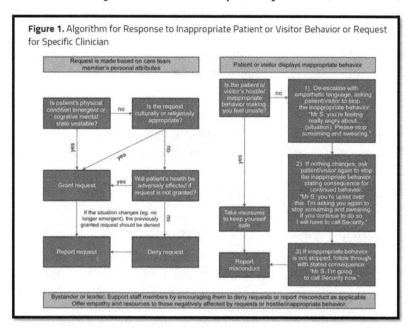

Figure 1. Algorithm for Response to Inappropriate Patient or Visitor Behavior or Request for Specific Clinician

The University of California at San Francisco (UCSF) uses a similar algorithm (Image 18) for reassigning patients with a focus on maintaining dignity of the affected minority health care workers and decreasing "moral distress and burnout."

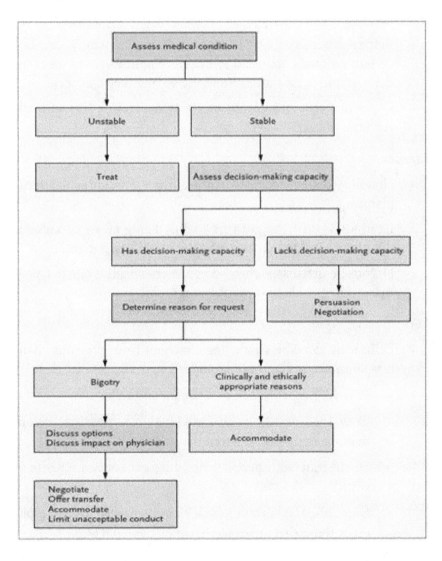

KNOWLEDGE, ATTITUDES, AND SKILLS

Knowledge

- Religion in and of itself is not linked to specific health disparities.

- Being a member of certain ethnic groups that tend to practice certain religions may lead to health inequities based on other demographic associations (and the setting they exist in).

- Issues that religious groups face may depend on their providers' level of bias.

Attitudes

- Handling patient requests requires nuance and organizational planning.

- I cannot say it enough times...while being aware of cultural differences and trends, focus on the individual patient!

- Do not be defensive when someone challenges your perspective on or attitude towards a demographic group.

Skills

- Utilize the same bias-reducing strategies from previous chapters to improve religious tolerance.

  - Practice perpetual self-assessment and reflection.

  - Treat each person as an individual; ask questions before making assumptions about them.

  - Spend time with people from different backgrounds than yours.

  - Learn about common health inequities in your field, especially those that are exacerbated by personal bias.

- Develop institutional policies and agreement on how to handle patient requests for their health care providers.

HOW TO TEACH ABOUT RELIGIOUS TOLERANCE

My favorite "ice breaker" for didactic sessions or trainings on religious tolerance is the administration of the Religious Literacy Quiz by Stephen Prothero of Boston University (Image 19). It can be distributed prior to your activity based on the "honor system," or you can allow your group up to ten minutes at the beginning of the meeting to complete the quiz. For residency programs, I split the physicians up by their year of training so that the interns, junior residents, and chief residents all compete against each other. They are allowed to work together in groups to complete the quiz, but there should be no use of cell phones, computers, or the internet to help find the correct answers.

The group's final answers should be written onto one page and turned in. For questions that have multiple answers, I give one point of credit for each correct answer, and I add up the total number of points (correct answers) to decide on the winner.

RELIGIOUS LITERACY QUIZ
STEPHEN PROTHERO, BOSTON UNIVERSITY

1. Name the Four Gospels. List as many as you can.

2. Name a sacred text of Hinduism.

3. Name the holy book of Islam.

4. Where, according to the Bible, was Jesus born?

5. George Bush spoke in his first inaugural of the Jericho road. What Bible story was he invoking?

6. What are the first five books of the Hebrew Bible or the Christian Old Testament?

7. What is the Golden Rule?

8. "God helps those who help themselves." Is this in the Bible? If so, where?

9. "Blessed are the poor in spirit, for theirs is the Kingdom of God." Does this appear in the Bible? If so, where?

10. Name the Ten Commandments. List as many as you can.

11. Name the Four Noble Truths of Buddhism.

12. What are the seven sacraments of Catholicism? List as many as you can.

13. The First Amendment says two things about religion, each in its own "clause." What are the two religion clauses of the First Amendment?

14. What is Ramadan? In what religion is it celebrated?

15. Match the Bible characters with the stories in which they appear. (Draw a line from one to the other; some characters may be matched with more than one story or vice versa.)

Adam and Eve	Exodus
Paul	Binding of Isaac
Moses	Olive Branch
Noah	Garden of Eden
Jesus	Parting of the Red Sea
Abraham	Road to Damascus
Serpent	Garden of Gethsemane

This activity helps the audience to see what their baseline understanding is of some of the major world religions. I often solicit feedback from participants about how they felt about their scores, and many of them are disappointed that they did not know more, including knowing more about the religions that they themselves practice. Stephen Prothero administered his quiz to almost 300 students over two years and had the following results for average scores, stratified by the religious affiliation of the quiz taker:

RELIGIOUS AFFILIATION	2006	2007
Catholic	50 percent	52 percent
Protestant	48 percent	44 percent
Jewish	38 percent	39 percent
Hindu/Buddhist/Sikh	34.5 percent	32 percent
Atheist/Agnostic	31 percent	26 percent

I typically share these results from Boston University so that my participants can see how they stack up against other groups of learners. But this activity does more than test someone's knowledge of other religions. By doing this activity together, especially in a diverse group, they are able to learn more about their colleagues who practice other religions. We have discussed the bias-reducing strategy of getting to know more about people from other backgrounds, and this is one way of doing so.

The explicit bias activity from Chapter 3 involving Juan Williams—I do not mean to keep picking on Mr. Williams, he just happened to give us a very useful example—can also be used during the session on religious tolerance. I often ask participants what they would have done if they were an institutional leader and a statement like the one that he made was said by a nurse, physician, staff member, supervisor, etc. I have already given examples of how to moderate that discussion.

Finally, I assess whether there are institutional policies on how to handle patient requests that are based on religion. If not, I like to use cases similar to the one presented in the bungle of the month to start off the discussion.

- Should obstetric call schedules be rearranged to accommodate patients who request female providers?
- Should outpatient clinic providers be asked to perform genitourinary exams for a male colleagues' patient if the patient requests it?

- What demographic requests from patients are acceptable? For example, is it okay to ask for a provider of a certain religion or a certain race?

If there are no organizational policies where I am presenting, I use the Mayo Clinic or UCSF algorithms discussed in this chapter as examples to demonstrate how they might institute guidelines to answer these questions.

¹Please see footnote below for comment regarding definitions of hijab and niqab

¹ Footnote #4: Definitions of hijab and niqab:

- *Hijab, niqab, and burka are coverings that are often worn by Muslim women and women of other religions as a sign of modesty.*
- *Hijab traditionally covers the head and neck area but leaves the face visible. This may be accomplished by the use of a simple headscarf.*
- *Niqab differs from hijab in that it also covers the majority of the face except for the area around the eyes.*
- *A burka conceals the entire face and body and often has a mesh covering to aid the wearer in seeing.*

CHAPTER 8

CULTURAL COMPETENCE VERSUS CULTURAL HUMILITY

Through a series of serendipitous events more than a decade ago, a group of medical students developed a relationship with seven communities in rural Honduras. The story is too long to rehash in its entirety, but it involved chance meetings between a medical student, their spouse who was doing field work in the Honduran mountains, and a local woman who married a Peace Corps volunteer. The result was the development of a public health organization with the goal of improving the health of women in those rural communities.

The initial needs assessments revealed a large burden of suffering from cervical cancer related to a lack of access to Pap smear screening. There was suitable infrastructure with adequate public health services available in the country, but the women in the rural mountain communities—where there was no electricity or running water at the time—did not have the resources or ability to commute to the major cities where they could receive cervical cancer testing. This lines up with international studies of low-resource countries that revealed screening rates as low as 5 percent.[1]

The medical students, who later teamed up with public health students from their same university, developed a system to assist the women in these small towns in obtaining the cervical cancer screening that was available in their country that they had been unable to receive. Through the use of head lamps, metal speculums, sterilizing supplies, small laboratory spatulas and brushes, glass microscope slides, and hair spray—that is correct, hair spray, look it up—the students recruited teaching physicians to collect cervical cytology specimens from the women in their communities. The physicians also received training in unaided visual inspection with acetic acid to expedite triaging of women who needed additional evaluation beyond cytology.

Unique medical record numbers were assigned for each woman, and the students transported the specimen slides to the capital city, Tegucigalpa, where they would be processed. This reduced the burden for women who had limited means to travel to other cities, and it did so at the very low cost of approximately $0.25 per person thanks to an affiliation agreement with la Asociación Hondureña de Planificación Familiar (Honduran Association for Family Planning, or "ASHONPLAFA").

In the second year of this partnership, I was asked to serve as one of the two faculty advisors for the trip, which I did that year and for the five years that followed. Because it involved students either performing service or receiving course credit, the school of medicine allowed me to spend the month in Honduras to supervise the project. This commitment involved a sign-up and scheduling week, followed by a rigorous one-week stretch of collecting hundreds of Pap smear specimens (averaging about 60-70 per day). During the one-week waiting period while they were being processed, we worked with lay health advisors to provide public health information and other services that had been requested during the previous year.

During the first year of the partnership (the year before I went), several women requested better family planning services and contraception, and the students went to work acquiring various methods of birth control. Through fundraising and donations, they developed a stockpile of oral contraceptive pills (OCPs), copper intrauterine devices (IUDs), and journal logs for natural family planning. When I joined the team the following year, I was rather surprised by the group's plans for delivering contraception in Honduras.

I was always under the impression that most Latin American countries had predominantly Catholic populations, so I figured that medical contraception such as the copper IUD would not be acceptable in Honduras. I had gotten to know several friends and coworkers who were Catholic, and some of them did not believe in using any type of birth control; the ones who did admitted to me that they would never notify their church members or family. The copper IUD is the most effective form of emergency contraception, and I had some Catholic patients who were particularly averse to that method.

At the time of my work in Honduras, more than half of the country's population was Catholic,[2] and I was nervous when I found out that the students had not notified anyone about their plans to provide contraception in the subsequent year—my first year there. I explained the potential to damage relationships and even be punished for providing forbidden services in a foreign country. I was also worried about making it through Customs with these medications and devices. This all occurred during a time when internet service was sparse in the region of the country we were going to, and the organizations that we worked with did not have websites. The students were disappointed, and they made plans to scrap the idea of providing contraception; all except for a few of them.

Fortunately, some of the students did not give up, and they made international phone call after international phone call, even discussing our proposal with officials from the ministry of health. It turns out that they were enthusiastic about our plans, and they offered to give us additional copper IUDs and OCPs to use. When the trip came, we actually held some of our public information sessions inside church buildings. There had been increasing national conversations in Honduras about the benefits of having smaller families, and the lay health advisors in the area were knowledgeable about the various methods of contraception. They were well-informed about side effects that require immediate attention, and they developed a system to assist women who needed removal of their IUD during the months that we were not in the country.

Although I still believe that I was correct in suggesting that we check with government officials (and Customs) about our plans for transporting and providing contraception in another country, I was overly confident that there was a problem where one did not actually exist. If not for the few vigilant students who spent hours investigating my concerns, we could have disappointed several communities and hundreds of families by not providing what they had requested the previous year.

I made a mistake that I have warned about in this book by stereotyping a nation of people without checking to see if the communities that we were working with shared the same beliefs as the Catholics I had met in the United States. I attempted to embrace the ideals of the previous chapter and practice religious tolerance through respect for the beliefs of others without checking to be sure that they held these beliefs. This small bungle of the month demonstrates the theme of this chapter—the problem with attempting to practice cultural competency without also being culturally humble.

DEFINITIONS

The concept of *culture* is defined by the Task Force on Community Preventive Services as patterns of thoughts and behavior that distinguish certain social groups from others.[3] In Chapter 6, we introduced a definition of *cultural competence* based on the work by Drs. Tervalon and Murray-Garcia that includes "inquiring about, responding to, and respecting beliefs and desires, regardless of the patient's age, gender, religion, ethnicity, or language."[4]

In the bungle of the month above, I had inquired about the reproductive health beliefs of my Catholic patients, I respected their requests for family planning services, and I responded to their desires without passing judgment. However, the missing piece was to be sure that other members of these groups shared the same beliefs as the majority of the people with whom I interacted. *Cultural humility* is an added approach to cultural competence that acknowledges the need for life-long learning as you will never be able to predict the beliefs and values of everyone that you meet.[5] Like we have discussed in Chapters 2 and 3 when we discussed confronting bias, self-reflection is a practice that can make us aware of our assumptions, stereotypes, and prejudices. Being culturally humble means focusing on and eliminating these negative behaviors and attitudes, which will help to address the power imbalances in the doctor-patient relationship.

CULTURAL INCOMPETENCE IN HEALTHCARE

Years ago, I was speaking to a perinatologist—a high risk obstetrician with fellowship training in maternal-fetal medicine—who had spent a large amount of time in his career on the L&D units of his hospitals. He works closely with anesthesiologists who provide regional anesthesia, commonly known as epidurals, for women who are in labor or undergoing a cesarean section. One day he had an interaction with an anesthesiologist who was caring for a mutual patient who spoke Spanish and had little English proficiency. The patient was not getting good pain relief from her epidural, so the anesthesia consultant was called back to check on things. He re-dosed her with a bolus of medication and appeared to be annoyed when they called him back a while later to address the patient's persistent, uncontrolled pain.

The L&D nurse and the perinatologist asked if there might be an issue with the epidural catheter placement, and the anesthesiologist replied that he doubted it because the problem is probably "supratentorial." For any non-clinicians who are reading this, saying that something is supratentorial means that it occurs above the tentorium cerebelli of the brain; in other words, it is a euphemism (typically used as a pejorative) for saying that something is not real but is "just in someone's head." When questioned why on Earth he would say that, he replied, "Most Hispanic women don't even ask for epidurals, so the fact that she wanted one in the first place means she might have something going on."

I apologize for not giving the juicy details of what ensued, but in the interest of time just know that it ended with a very apologetic anesthesiologist. He appeared to be contrite and said that he had been inappropriate with his language, but he did not back down from his experience that most of his Latina patients did not get epidurals.

The danger of this type of interaction should be obvious when a patient of a certain ethnicity is viewed by a physician as having a mental health problem just because they asked for medication for pain control while giving birth. This is reminiscent of our discussion in Chapter 3 that some medical students had already formed ideas that there were racial differences in how people perceive pain, and how Hispanic children were 28 percent less likely to receive opioid pain medication for the same types of long bone fractures as other children. But was our anesthesiologist's experience based in reality?

In studies of regional anesthesia in obstetric care, it is true that women who identify as Hispanic/Latina were less likely to use neuraxial analgesia such as epidurals compared to other groups—66 percent of primarily Spanish-speaking women versus 75 percent for English-speaking women.[6] Women's original plans for anesthesia showed an even greater disparity with a 30 percent difference; in other words, Hispanic women were much more likely to verbally decline epidurals during their prenatal care, but a significant number did change their mind once they were in labor. Implementation of educational interventions does not seem to change this significantly, so the trends that are seen are not likely due to a lack of health literacy.[7,8]

Not to beat up on my anesthesia colleague, but this even further demonstrates how problematic his way of thinking can be. He probably saw himself as a culturally competent physician who was aware of ethnic disparities in the use of neuraxial analgesia. However, he lacked the cultural humility to know that every Latina woman on the planet is not the same, and they are allowed to be different in how they address their pain. The fact that so many Hispanic women change their mind means that his type of thinking could miss women who initially decline anesthesia pain control but would later want it when their pain worsens.

Another related example occurred while I was rounding in the newborn nursery—the same place where I discovered my past implicit bias against people who smoke cigarettes (see Chapter 2 for details). This time, we were preparing to discharge a one-day-old Latino neonate whose mother had recovered quite well and declined to stay until the second postpartum day. I asked our resident physician team if the family wanted to have their son circumcised, and they gave me a very hesitant response of, "Uhhhhhhh…no."

I could sense that they might be guessing, so I asked them if they were sure they had remembered to ask. My resident gave me a response that was much kinder but still similar to the one from our anesthesiologist above. They told me, "Our Hispanic patients never get circumcisions for their sons." They had not read this book yet, so I gave them a pass and told them that we still needed to ask to be sure. We went in the room so that I could perform my final exam on the baby, and I asked the parents if they wanted the baby to receive a circumcision. I gave them my usual talking points about the risks and benefits of the procedure, but they ultimately declined. When we left the patient's room my resident said, "I told you so," and we all shared a good laugh.

Similar to the data about epidural anesthesia, my resident's experiences and expectations were somewhat supported by the data. In population level studies of race and ethnicity, the circumcision rates are 91 percent for White males, 76 percent for Black males, and only 44 percent for Hispanic males.[9] However, some of these differences are a result of cultural trends, but some of them are influenced by insurance coverage; circumcision rates are 24 percent lower in states that have lower Medicaid coverage for lower income patients. In previous years it was considered a cosmetic procedure, but the AAP shifted their stance on circumcision in 2012 based on several studies that demonstrated long-term benefits in the reduction of several infectious diseases.[10] They concluded that the incidence of benefits outweighed the incidence of risks at a ratio of approximately 100:1.

A *JAMA* study revealed that circumcision decreases the risk of HIV transmission by 60 percent, genital herpes transmission by 30 percent, and high-risk HPV transmission by 35 percent.[11] These data show the importance of being sure that patients decline a procedure, even if there are cultural trends that suggest that they might. It also raises the question of whether we should be more aggressive in trying to create cultural shifts in some interventions such as circumcision (e.g., when compared to use of regional anesthesia). Being culturally humble would encourage us to not try to change the culture of other people, but rather to offer the same high-quality care to everyone and allow patients to decide what is the best fit for them.

CULTURALLY COMPETENT AND CULTURALLY HUMBLE MEDICAL CARE AND MEDICAL EDUCATION

Cultural humility requires effective communication, shared decision-making, and respect for patient preferences. Good communication is more likely with the use of interpreters or bilingual providers whenever you are caring for patients who are non-native English speakers and would prefer to communicate in their native language. Similarly, patient information—including patient handouts—should be provided through culturally and linguistically appropriate services (CLAS). Several decades ago, the concept emerged of a competent community that could identify cultural needs and problems, reach a consensus on priorities, and agree on the ways of implementing change.[12] In the setting of health equity, this requires collaboration between healthcare organizations and cultural groups in the community. As president of the Academy of Family Physicians of India (AFPI), Dr. Raman Kumar and colleagues described five stages of organizational cultural competence, increasing chronologically from least to most desirable:[13]

1. Cultural destructiveness
2. Cultural incapacity
3. Cultural blindness
4. Cultural pre-competence
5. Cultural competence and proficiency.

In the early stages, healthcare organizations either lack the capacity or the will to provide culturally competent care, and they expect patients to adapt to their system. Cultural blindness creates a "one size fits all" type of system that is not aware of the unique needs of some of their patients. Culturally competent and culturally proficient institutions will have services that are convenient for a diverse patient population, involve community members and patients on advisory boards, and provide ongoing training and self-assessment as a means of quality improvement.

We previously discussed that the use of institutional paradigms to create system change is one way of overcoming individual behaviors that are biased or that lack cultural competence and humility. Since I often speak at academic medical centers, the AAMC paradigms have been very useful for me to demonstrate how this might be done. The AAMC and American Hospital Association describe the health, social, and business benefits of culturally competent healthcare organizations.[14] Culturally competent medical centers are more efficient, increase cost savings, reduce disparities in preventive care, and increase trust and respect with the community. With regard to culturally responsive education and training, the AAMC reported four key strategies:

1. Use evidence-based information based on scientifically rigorous literature.

2. Set specific, measurable, attainable, relevant, and time-based (SMART) goals. Examine cultural competence education within the IOM framework that we have used in this book of "Knowledge, Attitudes, and Skills."

3. While designing cultural competence curriculum, also consider and develop both qualitative and quantitative assessment and evaluation methods. This will be more effective if academic medicine faculty respond to the needs of patients and their communities and if the faculty are accountable for outcomes. (Think back to when we discussed academic department requirements to identify and eliminate health inequities within their field.)

4. Use methodologically rigorous evaluation tools to demonstrate curricular effectiveness.

HEALTH EQUITY

The AAMC's Cultural Competence Education and Training Assessment Inventory (CCETAI) and Tool for Assessing Cultural Competence Training (TACCT) are examples that provide rigorous, evidence-based guidance on the assessment component described above. The five TACCT domains include (1) defining cultural competence and related terms, (2) listing the key components of cultural competence, (3) understanding the harms of stereotyping and bias, (4) understanding the history of and underlying factors behind health disparities, and (5) development of cross-cultural clinical skills. The full AAMC document on cultural competence includes other valuable resources and recommendations for providing training in cultural competence, including the six-step approach to curriculum development described by Lipsett and Kern (Image 20).

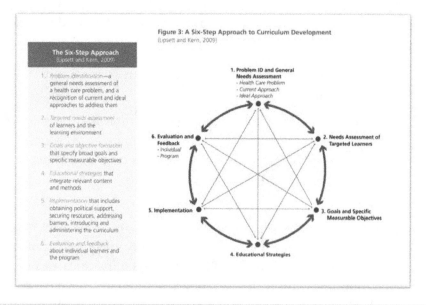

KNOWLEDGE, ATTITUDES, AND SKILLS

Knowledge

- Culturally competent health care providers and organizations learn about and respond to the beliefs and needs of particular cultural groups.

- Culturally humble people are culturally competent, but they also consider that everyone within a cultural group does not have the same principles, values, and desires.

- While cultural humility is the ultimate goal, learning about cultural trends can create an inclusive environment within your healthcare organization or academic center and uncover systemic biases.

Attitudes

- You will never be able to learn everything about other cultural groups, no matter how much time you spend around them.

- It is not even possible to know everything about all of the different types of people within your *own* cultural groups.

- Even within certain cultural groupings, there is significant heterogeneity within that group.

- Most countries will exhibit regional differences in trends, states and provinces will demonstrate high variability from city to city, and neighborhoods within a city may be very different from each other.

Skills

- Self-reflection is not only helpful for addressing bias, but it can also highlight stereotyping of certain cultural groups that masquerade as culturally competent care.

- On an individual level, learning cultural trends is important and might help you understand patients better...however, treat each person as a unique human being.

- Find the middle ground between overgeneralizing and cultural ignorance.

- If someone accuses you of not being culturally sensitive in a particular area, don't be offended...be humble, and ask them to help you understand.

HOW TO TEACH ABOUT CULTURAL COMPETENCE AND CULTURAL HUMILITY

Many of the cases and exercises from Chapter 7 on religious toler-ance are good ways to discuss cultural competence (e.g., the Stephen Prothero quiz) and cultural humility (e.g., how to address patient re-quests or preferences that are based on their religion). The AAMC materials for developing cultural competence curricula are available for free online from the AAMC website in portable document format (PDF). I have also had success by having discussions about the follow-ing two cases, which are based on real-life encounters that I have had with patients. As with all other clinical scenarios, certain details from the case are changed to protect patient privacy and confidentiality, and some of the cases are hybrids of several encounters.

CASE #1

A sixty-two-year-old woman is here for her annual physical in De-cember without any specific complaints. She has no active medical issues and has no past medical history except an appendectomy as a young adult. She is not currently taking any medications and has no known drug allergies. She works at a local mail and shipping compa-ny, and she identifies as an African American woman (see Chapter 4 if you are wondering why this was not included in the opening line of the case). Your patient is from rural South Carolina originally, but she has been living in your city for more than thirty years. She rides her bike for thirty to forty minutes per day and follows a primarily pescatarian diet. She has an unremarkable physical examination, is up to date on all of her cancer screenings, and the fasting labs that she obtained prior to her visit were all normal.

For her plan of care, you recommend an influenza vaccine and encourage her to continue her healthy lifestyle. She tells you that she does not trust vaccines, as they are an attempt to either poison Black people or insert something into their bodies. She has heard about things such as the Tuskegee Syphilis Experiment, so she would prefer natural methods of prevention that she can do on her own.

Cultural humility discussion point

- How do you address her concern about the influenza vaccine in a culturally humble way?

Cultural competence discussion point

- What do you do if you suspect that a future/different patient has similar concerns? For example, if another one of your Black patients has vaccine hesitancy, do you preemptively initiate a discussion about mistrust of the healthcare system?

CASE #2

This case is based on the bungle of the month from Chapter 6. It involves a man in his late teens or early twenties presenting for an annual physical prior to returning to college. He has no active medical issues and has a normal exam. He is a cisgender Black man from the town that you practice in. He mentions doing very well academically his freshman year, and as a result of studying so much he has not had time for a boyfriend.

You remember hearing that the lifetime risk of acquiring HIV infection for gay Black men in the United States is projected to be as high as one in two if things continue as they currently are (compared to one in ninety-nine for all Americans combined).

Cultural humility discussion point

- How do you counsel this patient while being culturally humble?

Cultural competence discussion point

- Are you practicing cultural competence by recognizing that your patient might have a higher risk of HIV if he has sex with men? Or is this just stereotyping?

Remember there are no "right or wrong" answers to these cases; they should be used as discussion points so that you can practice utilizing some of the institutional and individual methods for how to approach these complex situations.

CHAPTER 9

SOCIAL DETERMINANTS OF HEALTH AND HOMELESSNESS

DR. BONZO'S BUNGLE OF THE MONTH:
Unhoused ≠ Unemployed

Since 2017, my outpatient clinical work has been at an FQHC that also serves as a designated healthcare for the homeless (HCH) site. When I was in high school, I remember my parents having an interest in helping people who did not have stable housing, and they have served on the board of a local homeless shelter for many years. In my first year of medical school—which I cannot believe was almost twenty-five years ago—I often told people that I had an interest in providing primary care for homeless populations, although I did not know what that type of a career would look like.

Things fell into place five years ago when our nonprofit hospital system formed a partnership with my current HCH site, and I began to provide outpatient care there along with the other family medicine residency faculty. We were initially brought in to provide prenatal care and to perform gynecological procedures following the departure of their OB/GYN, but our residency director expressed interest in staffing their mobile homeless clinic.

When our hospital was bought by a for-profit private system, I left my role as a core faculty member and assumed a role as a community faculty member providing all my clinical care at the FQHC/HCH site. We have a brick-and-mortar clinic building, but our advanced practice providers, our resident physicians, and I also provide mobile clinical services every week at rotating sites around town. These locations include homeless camps (what some people refer to as tent cities), soup kitchens, and central locales that are close to areas with a high density of the patient population that we serve.

The mobile clinic staff is comprised of an interdisciplinary team that includes physicians, nurses, medical assistants, social workers, psychiatrists, homeless outreach coordinators, and the Homeless Authority. We started out providing acute, chronic, and preventive care, but the recent pandemic has caused us to add additional services. We now provide testing for SARS-CoV-2 as well as COVID-19 immunization with the three vaccines that are currently commercially available in the United States.

During one of my first times providing care at the mobile homeless clinic, I saw a well-dressed and clean-cut young man who looked like he was in the wrong place. He inadvertently skipped past the short triage line, walked up to me, and asked if we would be able to treat his seasonal allergies. I explained to him that this was a mobile clinic for homeless people, although we do have a clinic building where he is welcome to establish care. He informed me that he was indeed homeless and that he was staying at the shelter that we were stationed at on that day.

That was stereotype #1: I had an image ingrained in my head of homeless people being disheveled and frequently unshaven or with long hair.

I apologized and told him that he could step over to the triage line and that we would see him shortly. He was able to get registered, his clinical presentation was consistent with seasonal allergic rhinitis, and we treated him with the appropriate medication from our mobile unit. During the evaluation, he mentioned that he would like to get fasting blood work done to evaluate for diabetes or high cholesterol, because he has a family history of both conditions. I told him that we did not have the capacity to perform venous blood draws at our mobile clinic yet, but that we could set up an appointment at our clinic building location for his labs. I told him that the social worker would provide him with a bus pass so that he could get to our clinic site, but he declined, saying that he would just drive his car.

That was stereotype #2: I assumed that people who were chronically homeless or living in shelters would not be able to afford a car. I had heard stories of families briefly living out of their cars, but I did not think of an individual young man doing so. I differentiated someone living solo versus someone living with family while homeless.

I asked him what he did with his car when he was staying at the shelter to prevent it from receiving parking tickets or being broken into. He said that he had developed an arrangement with someone nearby who did not mind his car being left on their property. Given that he had convenient transportation, I directed him to our scheduling and registration team and asked them to schedule a follow-up lab appointment. Since he had a car, I told them that they could schedule him any time of the day, however he asked if we had any late hours. It turns out that we do, as our clinic stays open until 7:00 p.m. on certain days of the week. He mentioned how beneficial that would be because he works from 8:00 a.m. until 5:00 p.m. on most weekdays.

That was stereotype #3: I did not check to see what his weekly schedule was, because I did not have an image of a person living in a shelter as having a typical "9-to-5" job.

As the saying goes, "three strikes and you're out," so that is enough stereotyping for this chapter. In summary, this book should have demonstrated so far that implicit biases can extend to any historically marginalized or excluded group of people. We have discussed biases against smokers, women, young people using electronic devices, sexual and gender minorities, Black men, and religious minorities. So, it should not be surprising that I would have implicit biases against people experiencing homelessness, and I am sure that many people harbor explicit biases towards them as well.

Fortunately, this encounter happened in the first days of my work at the HCH mobile clinic, so I realized early on the importance of recognizing the diversity and heterogeneity of the homeless population.

In the five years since then, I have had the opportunity to get to know a wide range of people who bring with them a wide range of personalities and experiences. Now, I am no longer surprised by anyone that I meet in one of the camps, shelters, or soup kitchens. What is more important is recognition of the social needs and the barriers that exist for them and that are common for most members of these communities.

DEFINITIONS AND INTRODUCTION TO SOCIAL DETERMINANTS

The *social determinants of health* are the non-biomedical factors that influence health outcomes, such as socioeconomic status, availability of safe housing, quality and level of educational attainment, access to high quality health care (which is often determined by employment), transportation accessibility, exposure to violence and stress, and social infrastructure.[1] Former surgeon general Dr. David Satcher recommended the use of a social determinants of health approach to reduce health inequities.[2] When we first introduced this concept in Chapter 4, we cited that the WHO described the social determinants of health as the "single most important determinant of one's health status."

This assertion is supported by the Los Angeles County Department of Public Health, whose regression models demonstrated that social and economic factors affect morbidity and mortality to a greater extent than biomedical determinants (Image 21).[3] They estimated that the social determinants contributed 40 percent, while health behavior (e.g., smoking) contributed 30 percent, clinical care contributed 20 percent, and the physical environment contributed 10 percent.

The actual impact of social determinants of health could be even higher than predicted given that some other categories such as health behavior can be heavily influenced by social factors. Think back to my father's cigarette use described in Chapter 2, which began in childhood while he was growing up around and working on tobacco farms.

Cigarette smoking is a health behavior, but social factors might influence who begins smoking and how long they continue to smoke.

A twelve-year-old boy whose parents smoke cigarettes, who tell him that the dangers of tobacco are overblown, and who offer him cigarettes, would obviously be predisposed to smoking. Years later as an adult, if this same boy did not have health insurance or a primary care provider, then it might be more difficult for him to quit smoking since he would have less access to pharmacotherapy or counseling services that could aid him in smoking cessation. Considering the social determinants of health add additional context to the importance of being non-judgmental in exploring the health decisions and health behaviors of patients.

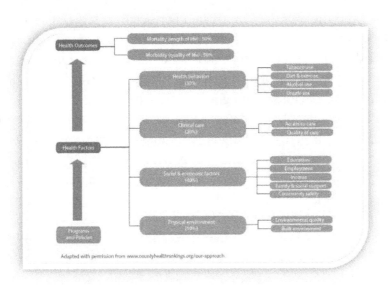

Adapted with permission from www.countyhealthrankings.org/our-approach.

In our previous discussion of race-based medicine, we laid out that the biological differences between races are often explained by social factors. In addition, research of racial health disparities sometimes fails to consider the impact of the environment on health outcomes. In Chapter 4, we explained how a race correction factor in spirometry (to measure pulmonary, or lung, function) is widely used without considering socioeconomic factors—such as pollution, or exposure to mold, dust, and cockroach allergens—that might affect the differences between races.[4,5] Project HOPE in Cincinnati, Ohio, demonstrated that housing code violations and increased density of housing units explained up to 22 percent of asthma-related ED visits.[6] In the same way that the quality of housing is an important social determinant that can have a major impact on morbidity and mortality, the absence of housing can have an even greater effect on health outcomes.

HOUSING AND HOMELESSNESS

We have placed heavy emphasis on definitions, wording, and the way we say things throughout this book. So many of the target groups that we have examined are subject to stigma in both their social and societal interactions (i.e., interpersonal interactions with individual people, and the way they are treated by society at large). Groups that suffer negative effects on their physical well-being are often simultaneously bombarded with negative mental and emotional messages that occur via the use of dehumanizing language towards them. Some examples are obvious; calling a homeless person a "bum" is agreed upon by most people to be unacceptable and mean-spirited. However, you might be surprised if you have not heard of some new trends, such as encouragement to move away from the word "homeless."

I have used the word homeless so far in this chapter as that is the language that is still traditionally used and recognized in society, and the alternatives are confusing for some people at times. In my day-to-day speech, I have found myself using the term less frequently, as I will explain below in just a moment.

The first time that I provided mobile health care in a homeless camp four years ago was also the first time that I had an up close and personal look at the living environment of a chronically homeless person. I was surprised by the vast differences in the residences in the community; some of them consisted of tarps that were tied around trees, while others were elaborate tents that looked like something a camping enthusiast would use. Regardless of the type of coverings that were used, several people had planted small flowers or other plants in an orderly fashion around their tents, and many of them had created a small walkway leading up to the entrance. The walkways were sometimes created by the orderly placement of rocks or gravel, and at other times someone had clearly tilled the ground to make a smooth pathway up to the entry of their home. That is correct, their *home*.

That is why some people, me included, are starting to use words such as *"houseless," "unhoused,"* or *"undomiciled,"* with the goal of eventually phasing out "homeless." Many people in these communities have homes, they just do not have houses, apartments, or permanent housing structures. Terms such as homeless do not distinguish between someone who is sheltered—either in a tent or in a local homeless shelter—from someone who is sleeping outdoors on a bench, unsheltered, or from someone who is sleeping in their car.

The distinct experiences of houseless people highlight a number of social determinants of health that affect this patient population.[7] A lack of consistent shelter can make medication storage difficult, especially for prescriptions like insulin that require refrigeration. Add to that a high incidence of severe financial constraints, and they often lack consistent food and water sources or access to transportation. Lack of transportation serves to further alienate them from a healthcare system where they sometimes feel that they are not welcome. They are at increased risk of physical and emotional abuse, as demonstrated in the Health Outcomes of People Experiencing Homelessness in Older Middle Age (HOPE HOME) Study.[8]

This prospective cohort study of older homeless adults showed that more than 10 percent of participants had experienced either violent or sexual victimization just in the prior six months alone. It is not surprising that they often resort to substance use and abuse to emotionally escape their world and numb some of the feelings associated with these circumstances. I still remember conversations about some of my patients' substance use, when they told me that was the only way they could cope with the reality that they were going out to the woods to sleep that night.

ADDRESSING SOCIAL DETERMINANTS OF HEALTH: HOUSING FIRST

The *Housing First Philosophy* is based on the belief that everyone is "housing ready," regardless of their life circumstances, substance use, or control of their mental health diagnoses. The *Housing First Model (HFM)* was initially developed for unhoused patients with dual diagnoses of substance abuse and serious mental illness; this typically represents 10–20 percent of homeless patients, although I have heard many people express an explicit bias that this is "the majority" of this population. The HFM does not have a sobriety requirement to obtain housing, and it has been shown to decrease substance abuse and its complications, to decrease ED visits and hospitalizations, and to decrease involvement in criminal activity.

The Downtown Emergency Service Center (DESC) in Seattle, Washington, describes two core principles of the HFM: "Housing is a basic human right, not a reward for clinical success," and "once the chaos of homelessness is eliminated from a person's life, clinical and social stabilization occur faster and are more enduring."[9] The DESC lists seven standards of a Housing First approach, which are summarized in an abbreviated manner below:

1. There should be no preconditions of accepting treatment (e.g., for substance abuse).

2. Housing should be accompanied by "robust support services" without any prerequisites.

3. Participation in these support services is not required to keep housing.

4. Target the most vulnerable and disabled homeless members first.

5. Use a *harm reduction approach* to addiction (more on this in Chapter 13).

6. Residents must have the same legal protections as any other tenants in the community.

7. Housing locations can be part of a "project-based or scattered site model."

An example of a "project-based model" in my current town is the Tiny House Project, which is a neighborhood that was constructed specifically for homeless Veterans (Image 22 below shows a group of our resident physicians in front of one of the model homes). One of the tiny homes in the entrance to the neighborhood was fashioned into a small clinic location for our FQHC/HCH, where a physician assistant provides care. During the COVID-19 pandemic, when regular clinic hours were difficult to establish, the Tiny House village was added to our list of locations served by our mobile clinic. The project-based model is convenient, as it provides a central location where clients and patients can access social services or medical care. However, a scattered site model could consist of random housing locations around the city that are eligible for Housing First, and it would still provide the benefits described above.[10]

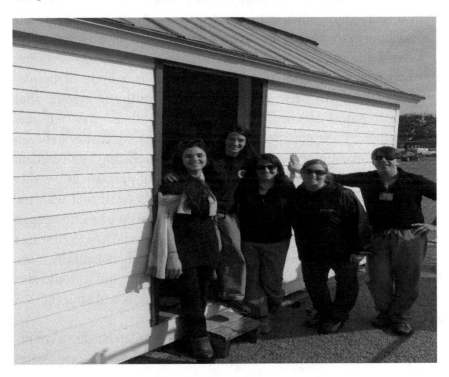

In addition to having better health-related and social outcomes, addressing the social determinant of housing is remarkably cost effective. The Denver Housing First Collaborative demonstrated an average cost savings of $31,545 on emergency services per person over two years ($15,773 per person annually).[11] A randomized controlled trial of 260 chronically homeless individuals in New York (Tsemberis and Stefancic, 2007) assigned participants to either a HFM pathway or to a control group of "treatment-as-usual" with the local county department of social services.[12] The majority of people in the HFM group maintained permanent, independent housing with cost savings up to $23,000 per person annually compared to care in homeless shelters.

The American Round Table to Abolish Homelessness (www.abolitionistroundtable.com) has also made the economic case for Housing First. Like the studies above, they have demonstrated that the use of public resources by chronically unhoused individuals—emergency medical services, hospitalizations, psychiatric treatment, law enforcement—is more expensive than the cost of housing (Image 23). More than seventy-five studies in the United States, Australia, and Canada have demonstrated the cost effectiveness of a Housing First approach.

The American Round Table to Abolish Homelessness describes the concept of "random ricocheting," which is a cycle of bouncing back and forth between accessing the healthcare system after significant illness sets in, and engagement with the law enforcement system. Their cost-benefit analyses estimate a cost of between $35,000–$150,000 per person for random ricocheting compared to only $13,000–$25,000 per person for the cost of permanent housing (Image 23). The lower end of these estimates is consistent with the studies in Denver and New York described above. When I first began to study this data, I questioned why society allows people to continue to live on the streets, knowing that it would not only holistically make their life better to provide them permanent housing, but it would also save society money. After discussions with friends and colleagues, I received my answer about why this happens.

One memorable interaction with a fellow physician led to a counter argument from them that the government frequently exaggerates or even lies about the costs of certain interventions. Even when the intention is not nefarious, my coworker gave examples of the government underestimating how expensive certain projects would be or the downstream costs that would occur as a result of implementation. When I explained that the Housing First studies were not performed by the government, then the conversation switched to reluctant acceptance about a potential small effect in a few carefully selected locations. My colleague doubted that this would work on a more widespread level, to which I showed them the numerous cost effectiveness studies in a wide variety of locations.

When I even showed them that this was effective in other countries that have different styles of government, a circular argument ensued that they did not trust the data about the cost savings. When it became obvious that they had never studied any data about homelessness, and that they could not provide any counter argument other than, "I don't believe you," I decided to stop wasting my time and ended the conversation.

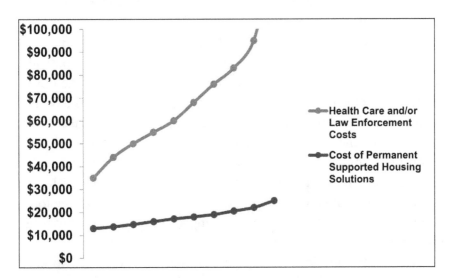

While studies in the United States, Australia, and Canada have demonstrated success using a Housing First approach at a local level, Finland has successfully implemented it at the national level.[13] In 2007, they set up a working group to address homelessness that resulted in the country setting up tens of thousands of *independent* apartments where people have the option of living alone. They used a *harm reduction model* that does not require participants to give up drug use but does offer substance abuse help if the person desires it. The Finnish model aims to build trust with clients, treats them as equals to the people providing the housing or other services, and tries to disrupt power imbalances in the relationship. Along with receiving permanent housing, the goal is to also help people integrate back into their communities via robust social networking and support.

Finland has a population of 5.5 million people, but only a few hundred are chronically undomiciled (i.e., living in shelters or on the street). Of the 0.1 percent of the population labeled as homeless, the overwhelming majority of them at least have temporary housing.

ADDRESSING OTHER SOCIAL DETERMINANTS OF HEALTH

One of the biggest hurdles in addressing the social determinants of health in clinical settings is convincing clinicians that it is their job to do so. Early in my career, I agreed with some of my teaching physicians who warned me to never give more effort than my patients did in improving their health. Hopefully, by this point of the book, you have rejected that way of thinking in the same way that I have for the past decade, with the understanding that a person's social context and life experiences influence their motivation and capacity to change health behaviors. Making an extra phone call to arrange for social services, filling out paperwork for medication assistance or housing, and developing an accessible resource with options for free food should be valued just as much as ordering a laboratory test or writing a prescription.

I have heard physicians complain that they feel like social workers on some days, but they might not be considering that these actions are probably more beneficial to decreasing the morbidity and mortality of their patients than any clinical care that they could provide (as we discussed at the beginning of this chapter). The ability to address poverty, housing, education, etc., is highly variable based on the setting that a clinician practices in. I am fortunate to work at a FQHC/HCH site that receives federal funding to assist us in taking care of patients who do not have health insurance or who are houseless. We have a dentist, eye doctor, psychiatrist, psychological counselor, and pharmacist on site; our patients can receive telehealth visits with a cardiologist or pick up their medications in our pharmacy either for free or for a significantly reduced price. This occurs in a city where other patients often have to wait months to see a psychiatrist or psychiatric nurse practitioner, or where uninsured patients often do not have access to specialists unless they are in the hospital.

Our organization employs social workers, Medicaid enrollment specialists, and community outreach coordinators, and we also have weekly collaborations with the local homeless authority, homeless advocates, and behavioral health specialists. A physician, nurse practitioner, or physician assistant in a small private practice might not have the capacity to hire some of the employees that work at a FQHC, so this highlights the importance of establishing interdisciplinary community partnerships at the individual provider and corporate levels.

Early in my medical career, I would dread the moments when patients told me they were being evicted from their home, or when they told me they were having difficulty affording food or clothes for their children. It was not that I lacked empathy for their situation, I just did not know how to help them. While working as a physician, I went back to school and became a part-time graduate student in a Master of Public Health (MPH) program. My thesis, completed in 2014, explored the barriers to collaboration between public health and primary care, which included the territorial nature of healthcare organizations.

In my fieldwork, I discovered a clinic that desperately needed nutrition services for their patients, but the providers in the clinic did not know the health department on the same street had some of these services available for free. Not only that, but the health department was disappointed with the poor attendance and engagement in some of their programs. I realized that there are typically numerous local public health and community medicine organizations that address the social determinants of health, but clinicians are often not aware of them. Even when they were aware of them, I often encountered hesitancy to allow "outsiders" into their clinic and hospital walls to help patients.

Over time, I noticed trends in the social needs of my patients. And as time went on, I became comfortable telling patients, "I don't have the answer, but let me see if I can find someone who does." This eventually led to a coalition of people and organizations that provide services to aid patients with housing problems, food insecurity, and limited health literacy. When I began working for the FQHC/HCH, this coalition became even more robust because of the infrastructure that already existed. The social determinants that are most critical to address are going to vary by geographic location.

For example, in Brooklyn, New York, an emergency room physician (and former classmate of mine) named Dr. Robert Gore noticed the devastation that gun violence was having on his community, so he started the Kings Against Violence Initiative (https://www.kavibrooklyn.org), which mobilized the community to provide youth violence intervention programs in hospitals and schools.

The United States healthcare system reimburses clinical organizations for medical care that they provide, but a shift towards additionally reimbursing for social interventions would encourage clinicians to address these important determinants of health. Also, healthcare organizations should be bold and invest in programs that may cost money up front but will be cost effective downstream.

KNOWLEDGE, ATTITUDES, AND SKILLS

Knowledge

- The social determinants of health are the non-biological factors that influence health outcomes.

- Social determinants of health have a more significant impact on morbidity and mortality than clinical care or other biomedical determinants of health.

- Housing is arguably the most important social determinant of health.

- Providing housing for people experiencing chronic homelessness improves their health outcomes, including improvement in their mental health and decrease in complications from substance abuse.

Attitudes

- Do not be afraid or intimidated to address the social determinants of health. This is one of the best ways that you can be an advocate for patients.

- Everyone is housing ready, regardless of their drug use or mental health diagnoses; this is a Housing First approach.

- Housing First not only improves outcomes for individuals, but it is also cost effective to society.

Skills

- For healthcare organizations, facilitate community partnerships and allow public health organizations increased access to your patient populations. Stop being so territorial!

- Also, for healthcare organizations, financially support initiatives that provide or build housing for people experiencing chronic homelessness.

- For individual clinicians, prioritize locating community partners to assist you in addressing complex social determinants such as housing.

- For medical educators, blend the teaching of pathophysiology and medical management with the social determinants of health.

- Utilize a Housing First approach in your advocacy to address homelessness.

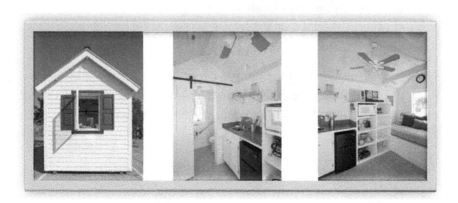

HOW TO TEACH ABOUT SOCIAL DETERMINANTS OF HEALTH

Whenever I am giving an academic lecture or consulting talk, my introduction typically encourages the audience to ask questions as we go. Active learning and crowd interactions tend to hold the participants' attention and enhance the retention of information, and it also ensures that no one is confused by the topics being discussed. When I was once giving a Grand Rounds presentation on housing and the social determinants of health, I was barely a minute into my presentation before a man in the last row raised his hand; this was not out of the ordinary except that it occurred so early in the session. I called on him and he proclaimed, "We have to decide if we are going to raise a generation of physician scientists or if we are just going to train a bunch of social workers."

I remained calm and began to tell him that there is a need for both social workers and physicians, and that my talk on that day would describe the importance of interdisciplinary collaboration between the groups. I then started to say that addressing the social determinants of health and clinical care should be integrated, but he stood up and started walking out before I could even finish my sentence. The topic of my talk was clearly outlined on the flyer at the auditorium entrance, so he could not have been surprised by my topic. It seemed that he came that morning just to make that statement and leave in protest.

After my presentation, several people apologized and said that the man from earlier was a community physician who sometimes shows up to department presentations to make negative comments; they dismissed him as a "troll." One of the resident physicians later told me that the disgruntled audience member was simply parroting a talking point from a former faculty member at the Perelman School of Medicine at the University of Pennsylvania. Dr. Stanley Goldfarb published an op-ed in the *Wall Street Journal* that mocked the teaching of social justice issues in medical school, such as appropriate pronoun use for sexual and gender minorities. (In case anyone feels that I am editorializing, the title of his article was, "Take Two Aspirin and Call Me by My Pronouns.")[14] He bemoaned the newfound interest in "eliminating health disparities" and teaching cultural competency, fearing that this would interfere with the teaching of "medical science."

If Dr. Goldfarb had been fortunate enough to read this book (particularly this chapter and Chapter 4) before writing his editorial piece, he would have realized two things: (1) eliminating health disparities and addressing social issues actually improves outcomes on a much greater scale than "medical science" and (2) a lot of the medical and scientific issues that he would rather we focus on are caused by social factors and can be prevented by addressing the social determinants of health. *This should be your focus when teaching about the social determinants of health,* and this is the main reason that I shared my Grand Rounds story here. (The secondary reason was so that you can be prepared for some members of your audience who do not feel that this chapter is in the purview of medical education.)

Although the topics from this book can be taught to your target audience in any order, *I strongly recommend that you cover Chapter 4 with your learners prior to undertaking the teaching points from this chapter.* I learned that an understanding of the limitations of race-based medicine is important to prevent your audience from believing that certain racial and ethnic health disparities are simply caused by differences in genetics. Once they understand that most health inequities are caused by social factors, they will be more open to accepting their role in addressing the social determinants of health.

The case on cardiovascular disease presented at the end of Chapter 4—which explained why being Black is more dangerous than smoking—pairs well with this discussion. We previously explained that the differences in hypertension among African Americans are related to diets that are higher in calories and sodium but lower in potassium, paired with higher rates of sedentary living and higher exposure to stress.[15] This is a good opportunity to discuss how food deserts, community violence, and lack of economic opportunity contribute to hypertension. You can also begin discussions of how you and your healthcare organizations can overcome these barriers. For undergraduate medical education, teaching the social determinants of health at the same time that you teach these medical topics will make them feel less distinct from each other.

CASE

For more clinically oriented discussions on how a physician or advanced practice provider would address social factors at the point of care, I have utilized the following case:

- History of present illness: forty-eight-year-old man was admitted to the hospital with dizziness, blurry vision, and mild confusion. (If you want to know his race at this point, go back and reread Chapter 4.)

- Past medical history: hypertension, type 2 diabetes mellitus (last hgb A1c 14.6 percent) with multiple hospital admissions for hyperosmolar hyperglycemic nonketotic coma

- Current medications: metformin 1000mg twice daily, lisinopril 40mg daily, triamterene/hydrochlorothiazide 75mg/50mg daily

- Social history: non-smoker, currently living in a homeless encampment that is approximately six miles from the hospital

164

- Vital signs: blood pressure 158/96, pulse 123, respiratory rate 20, temperature 36°C

- Pertinent physical exam findings: disheveled/unkempt, heart is rapid but has a regular rhythm, borderline tachypnea but no rhonchi or wheezes, poor capillary refill

- Pertinent labs: glucose 799mg/dL, sodium 151 mEq/L (normal 135-145), bicarbonate 18 mEq/L (normal 22-29), serum osmolality 325 mOsm/kg H_2O, arterial blood gas pH 7.32

At this point, you can use this case to review the diagnosis of medical management of hyperosmolar hyperglycemic nonketotic coma, and to differentiate it from the clinical presentation and treatment of diabetic ketoacidosis. As you finish discussing the medical management, continue with the discussion on addressing the social determinants of health.

- Hospital Course:

  1. Patient was placed on an insulin drip for a day and had resolution of his metabolic encephalopathy with improvement in his hyperglycemia.

  2. He was transitioned to subcutaneous (SC) insulin the following day and maintained normal glucose levels.

  3. The patient's diet was advanced, his intravenous fluids were discontinued, and discharge planning was initiated.

  4. He was prescribed the following new medications: glargine insulin thirty-five units injected SC at bedtime, aspart insulin ten units SC with meals.

- When you tell him that he is being discharged, the patient asks if he can stay an extra night because it is very cold and there is a thunderstorm outside.

Points for Discussion:

- If you are a resident physician or advanced practice provider, would you ask your attending physician to let him stay another night?

- If you are the attending physician, would you try to let him stay for another night?

- If you are a hospital administrator, would you allow the medical team to let him stay another night, knowing that the extra day would not likely be reimbursed by Medicaid? (Or if the patient is uninsured, would you allow him to stay another night knowing that there will be hospital costs that you are unlikely to recover?)

- Where is he going to store his insulin? Is that your responsibility?

- Are you responsible for addressing his housing situation? If so, what steps would you take at this time?

CHAPTER 10

HEALTH INEQUITIES AFFECTING DISABLED/ DIFFERENTLY ABLED PEOPLE

DR. BONZO'S BUNGLE OF THE MONTH:
Slow Down

One nice thing about being a physician is that people always assume you are busy, which leads them to extend the benefit of the doubt and offer grace towards you when you are running late or appear to be preoccupied. In the early parts of my career, random pager alerts were acceptable reasons to step out of meetings to return a call, and in recent years pagers have been replaced by the ubiquitous cell phone.

As I have moved into senior leadership positions in my institution, I do not have the same freedom to show up late or step out of meetings to answer calls. I am sometimes the one running the meeting, and if not, there is a high probability that I will be called on by whoever is conducting the meeting. I try to maintain a high level of professionalism and I also want to respect the time of attendants, so I now abhor being late to events or meetings. Keep that in mind as I tell you about this chapter's bungle.

I was driving to an administrative meeting and was running "borderline" late. I knew how long it took to drive to work when there was typical traffic, and the time that I was leaving meant that I would be on time only if I did not have any surprises. Fortunately, there was not a lot of traffic, but I needed to make most of the stoplights or else I was going to be tardy. Traffic was slightly congested as I approached the final major intersection before work, but I knew that I would make it on time if I could make it through this light without delay.

The two lanes of traffic appeared to be of equal length, so I was debating with myself whether I should stay where I was or change lanes. *Maybe I should get over into the left lane in case someone in the right lane slows up to make a turn. No wait, I would feel really stupid if I switched lanes and it was slower than the one that I'm in.* More cars were approaching from behind, so I needed to make a quick decision.

I looked up and the car in front of me had a wheelchair insignia on the license plate tag, so I reflexively moved over into the other lane. The car that I pulled behind was operated by a driver who was looking down at something, maybe a cell phone, so I had to honk to get him to start driving. He began driving at a normal speed, which was nowhere near the pace of the car with the handicap placard, which definitely pulled away going quite a bit above the speed limit. You can probably guess how the story ends; the car in front of me missed the light (and thus, by default, so did I), while the car with the handicap placard and several cars behind it easily made it through. And yes, I was about two minutes late to my meeting, which is the exact length of time that I had to wait at that red light.

At this point of the book (or really at any point beyond Chapter 2), you can probably psychoanalyze me and guess exactly what contributed to my behavior on that day. I had a bias that the car with the handicap placard would be slower than other cars. This was clearly linked to a stereotype that I had about the people who drive such cars. It happened so quickly that I did not have time to acknowledge it until it was too late, but once it occurred, I immediately realized what I had done.

If you had asked me before that day whether I had an explicit bias that people driving cars with handicap placards are slow, I would have told you "No." But neither car was older or dirtier, neither one looked like a sports car, and both cars were about the same size. There was only one thing that stood out or that differentiated those two cars, which was the license plate with the wheelchair symbol.

After hearing this story, you probably agree that a bias was definitely present within me at the implicit, or unconscious, level. It rose to the explicit level very quickly, and it caused me to be late to my meeting. In addition, if I had made the stop light, it might have reinforced an ugly stereotype in my brain.

This anecdote sets the stage for this chapter's discussion about disabilities, which is susceptible to the same forces that create inequities for the other target groups that we have discussed so far in this book. They are a diverse group of people with different health care needs and different experiences, but they do have some shared experiences with regard to the societal and systemic barriers that are common in their lives. We all have some preconceived notions about people living with disabilities, we all have preferences for or against them, and we need to make system changes to overcome these biases and to ensure that members of this community have the opportunity to achieve health equity.

DEFINITIONS AND TERMINOLOGY

By now, I have hopefully convinced you that words matter, so let us discuss the good, the bad, and the ugly regarding the terminology used in discussing disabilities. First, starting with the word *disabled*, I noticed several years ago that more people were using the term *"differently abled"* in place of disabled. A particular guest speaker in one of my graduate school courses was very assertive in telling us that we should no longer use the word disabled. His point of view was that the root *dis* was Latin for "the opposite of," so calling someone disabled was saying that they were "the opposite of able." He contended that some people are just different, but that they are still valuable contributors to society and able to accomplish great things, hence his preference for the term differently abled.

In more recent years, I came across an article in the *HuffPost* by Zachary Fenell entitled, "Stop Saying 'Wheelchair Bound' and Other Outdated and Offensive Terms to People with Disabilities."[1] In the article, he does not feel that the terms "disabled" or "handicap" are inappropriate, but he does feel that using the term "wheelchair bound" is outdated and potentially offensive. He offers up potential alternative ways to discuss disabilities, as outlined in the table below.

POTENTIAL ALTERNATIVE TERMINOLOGY AND LANGUAGE WHEN DISCUSSING DISABILITIES	
Commonly Used Term	*Potential Replacement Term*
Wheelchair bound	Wheelchair user
Handicap vehicle	Wheelchair accessible vehicle
Sufferer/victim of disability	Living with disability
Handicapped	Disabled
Disabled	Differently abled

Zachary Fenell acknowledged the heterogeneity among disabled patients and made it clear that different people prefer different terminology. He recognized that these types of discussions sometimes feel like "trying to avoid the metaphorical tripwire," which creates the possibility that he considers certain terminology offensive but understands that not everyone will agree. The one exception that I have not heard any disagreement about is that the use of the word "r*tarded" to refer to people with intellectual or development disabilities is an offensive slur, and the informal shortening of this word is even more despicable.

In a footnote in the Preface, I discussed that some Hispanic Americans are choosing the term Latinx to refer to their ethnicity, while other Hispanic people feel that this term exemplifies an imperialistic attitude that seeks to anglicize foreign languages. The same phenomenon exists in this chapter; I once used the term "differently abled," and a wheelchair user lamented that doing so creates the impression that something is wrong with being disabled. Fenell questioned whether the use of the term "differently abled" could infer that people without disabilities do not differ from each other. I have met several people who agree with embracing the word disabled, so I have learned to stay patient and open my mind to different opinions.

In the *Knowledge, Attitude, and Skills* section of Chapter 3 and Chapter 7, I discussed the importance of not taking it personally when a member of a target group criticizes your language or perspective.

Try not to be defensive; use those moments as learning opportunities. Most importantly, when someone tells you how they would like to be referred to or says that they are offended when you use certain language with them, respect their wishes.

Since Chapter 3, we have placed a heavy emphasis on the importance of observing health inequities from a systemic viewpoint while still holding individual people accountable for their actions. We previously discussed how modern discourse often involves a debate about whether or not certain people are racist, but our health equity framework focuses on Dr. Jones' definition of systemic racism in examining how the current system structures opportunities based on social stratification by race.

Ableism at the individual level could be presented as discriminatory behavior towards disabled people or a view that they are inferior.[2] In his article on ableism in the medical profession, Dr. Shane Neilson uses a systemic viewpoint in discussing "practices or policies" that use able-bodiedness as the default in healthcare systems and treats disabled people as "invisible."[3] Fiona Kumari Campbell also discusses systemic bias as a "network of beliefs" that favors a certain typical "corporeal standard."[4] Campbell explains that the medical profession's biased paradigm for treating disabled people can also shape the way that society at large—including policymakers—view disability.

HEALTH INEQUITIES AMONG DISABLED/DIFFERENTLY ABLED PEOPLE

In Chapter 1, we summarized some of the health disparities that affect disabled populations in the United States.[5] Despite being four times more likely to report being in fair or poor health compared to other people, they receive unequal medical care by the healthcare system. They often avoid medical care because of an inability to afford health services, and they have a higher prevalence of chronic diseases. However, when they do present for medical care, they are less likely to receive the preventive services that are recommended by groups such as the USPSTF. Military veterans have rates of disability that are higher than the general population and combat-related injuries can lead to physical and mental health problems or cognitive impairment.

A few years ago, at a Starfield Summit conference, Bill Schwab discussed some of the various health inequities affecting disabled people, and he also discussed their treatment as a health disparities target group.[6] The life expectancy of men and women in the general population (based on sex assigned at birth) is 76.3 years and 81.1 years, respectively; for people with developmental disabilities (DD), the life expectancy is 59.9 years and 62.5 years for males and females, respectively. For people with intellectual disabilities (ID), they are more likely to miss cancer screenings, are less likely to receive vaccines on time, have poorer control of their chronic diseases, and are less likely to visit a dentist regularly. When they have poor vision, it is less likely to be detected in a timely manner.

People with ID are more likely to use psychotropic medications, many of which contribute to higher rates of obesity in this population; this creates a cycle, as the higher rates of obesity can worsen metabolic disorders that have a high incidence among people with disabilities. Given these significant inequities, I believe that disabled people should be treated as a medically underserved population (MUP), and they are obviously one of the target groups of this book; this is based not only on the disparities in outcomes that they experience but also on the systemic barriers that perpetuate these differences.

Health disparity populations, as defined by the National Association of State Directors of Developmental Disability Services (NASDDDS), support the inclusion of people with disabilities as a MUP. They define these populations as having "a significant disparity in the overall rate of disease incidence, prevalence, morbidity, mortality, or survival rates in the population as compared to the health status of the general population."[7] In addition to the evidence for disparities above, people with developmental disabilities have health care priorities that are frequently different than other people in the community. For example, the most common causes of death in the general population of the United States include atherosclerotic cardiovascular disease (heart disease and stroke), cancer, chronic lung disease (emphysema, asthma, and chronic bronchitis), and unintentional injury.[8]

For people with ID/DD, they also have high rates of heart disease and cancer, but the other leading causes of death include aspiration pneumonia, Alzheimer's disease, and septicemia.[8] Sepsis and other infectious diseases are sometimes not recognized in populations that may have limitations on their ability to communicate symptoms, or in people whose physical characteristics can hide certain physical findings. Bias among health care providers may lead to hesitation to perform a thorough examination for patients that are more time and labor intensive (this was discussed in Chapter 2).

By this point of the book, I hope that you are already thinking that, as with the other target groups discussed so far, people with disabilities represent a diverse, heterogeneous population. Every person with low vision will not have the same life experience, and some will have more barriers in health care depending on the nature or level of their disability. Studies of ableist microaggressions demonstrate a worse social experience when people have more visible disabilities or physical impairments.[9] You are also hopefully already considering the impact that intersectionality will have on the social experience of disabled people.

For example, a wheelchair user frequently faces challenges in community buildings that do not have functioning wheelchair-friendly doors, surfaces, or sidewalks. That wheelchair user will have other barriers besides ableism if they additionally have to face some of the individual and systemic biases discussed in this book, such as racism, sexism, homophobia, and xenophobia. For example, a qualitative study of almost 200 disabled sexual and gender minorities found that they experience unique microaggressions that are sometimes resistant even to social support; this population had lower satisfaction with LGBTQ+ support groups because of an ableist experience.[10]

COMBATING BIAS AGAINST DISABLED/DIFFERENTLY ABLED PEOPLE

In their health disparities consensus statement, the American Academy of Developmental Medicine and Dentistry (AADMD)—a nonprofit organization of interdisciplinary health professionals—discussed how people with neurodevelopmental disorders and intellectual disabilities (ND/ID) do not receive appropriate health promotion, preventive screenings, and medical surveillance.[11] Four of the main problems that they identify as contributing to the ableism seen in healthcare include:

1. Clinicians harbor limiting attitudes toward individuals with ND/ID, which contributes to stigma and marginalization.

2. Patients with ND/ID are rarely included in mainstream clinical trials.

3. Patients with ND/ID are not adequately transitioned from pediatric to adult-focused care.

4. The Health Resources and Services Administration (HRSA) does not recognize people with ND/ID as a MUP.

The AADMD offers up the following five suggestions as the most important ways to improve the situation:

1. People with ND/ID should be formally recognized as constituting a MUP.

2. Health education curricula should include opportunities to develop an understanding and appreciation of the unique qualities and rich opportunities possible for individuals with ND/ID.

3. Health care providers should adopt clinical guidelines, protocols, and best practices related to the health promotion, disease prevention, and specific treatment needs of patients with ND/ID.

4. Education of health care professionals should include knowledge of the movement towards community-based living, education, employment, socialization, person-centered planning, self-determination, and quality healthcare that reflects the desired experience of this population.

5. Many people with ND/ID need accommodations, support, and resources to do so successfully. Physicians, dentists, and other health care providers should strive to serve as health care advocates. (Commit to health parity and their highest quality of life possible.)

Zachary Fenell, mentioned earlier in this chapter, stresses the importance of using a person-first narrative that showcases the person first rather than their disability. For example, he said that he would prefer to be called "Zachary Fenell, an author with cerebral palsy," as opposed to "an author with cerebral palsy, Zachary Fenell." A parallel in healthcare would be to refer to "{patient name}, the patient admitted with a vaso-occlusive sickle cell pain crisis," as opposed to "the sickle cell patient in room 537." We should think about what kind of stereotypes we invoke when using certain language, such as when patients with sickle cell disease are described as "sicklers." This is not only dehumanizing language, but it can also create an image for a group that is frequently stereotyped as opioid abusers.

People with sickle cell disease have a life expectancy twenty-one years shorter than people without these disorders, and they also have rates of disability as high as 69 percent in some studies.[12,13] Add to this the fact that the majority of people with sickle disease in the United States are classified as African American, and you can imagine their intersectional experience of disability and race.

Our family medicine residency program's clinic has a sickle cell clinic that is supervised by family medicine attending physicians along with a hematology-oncology specialist. The residency inpatient service admits any of the patients in this clinic when they present to the hospital, and we have discussed compassionate care for patients who live with a painfully disabling disease. While we should be sure that individual clinicians are responsible for providing appropriate care and using appropriate language, we should also focus on addressing the system to create change—which has been described ad nauseum in this book so far.

In treating patients with sickle cell disease, instituting quality improvement initiatives that assess adherence to the National Heart, Lung, and Blood Institute (NHLBI) guidelines would be an important step for a hospital system.[14] For example, electronic medical record systems and ED policies could ensure that pain medications are administered within sixty minutes of registration or within thirty minutes of triage, as per the guidelines.

KNOWLEDGE, ATTITUDES, AND SKILLS

Knowledge

- Disabled people overall have worse medical outcomes in terms of mortality and prevalence of chronic disease, yet often do not receive the recommended standard of care in healthcare facilities.

- Differently abled or disabled patients are less likely to receive the same medical and dental preventive care as other patients. Stigma, implicit biases, and inconvenience may drive this.

- Disabled people are more likely to be affected by multiple social determinants of health compared to other populations, and higher rates of smoking or physical inactivity may also exacerbate health problems.

- As with the other target groups discussed so far, biases against patients with disabilities have the potential to cause harm, and so-called positive stereotypes can be infantilizing.

Attitudes

- It is important to be culturally competent _and_ culturally humble when providing health care for disabled patients.

- We should be aware of general trends regarding preferred terminology. (For example, some people prefer the term "disabled," while others prefer "differently abled.")
- Use a person-first narrative when discussing patients or clients living with disabilities; language should focus on the person, not their disability or disease process.
- Do not allow yourself to be offended if someone has a new or different preference in terminology or language than what you are used to...even if another disabled person told you that it was okay. Refer to that person in the way that they want to be referred to.

Skills

- Avoid media and settings that foster or encourage negative stereotypes.
- Spend time with people that are different than you. Many disabled people live in isolation, and increased interaction can be mutually beneficial.
- Utilize the skills discussed previously in being aware of differences and trends but treating each person as an individual.
- At the same time, make systemic changes to overcome ableism in healthcare.

HOW TO TEACH ABOUT DISABILITIES

Bill Schwab's speech at the Starfield Summit, which was referenced earlier in the chapter, is an excellent, concise video that lends itself well to initiating a discussion about health disparities among disabled people. It is only about eight minutes long and can be played at the beginning of your sessions on disabilities, or it can be distributed to your audience to be viewed ahead of time. I have utilized the following questions, inspired by the Starfield Summit presentation, to spark dialogue during my didactic and consulting sessions on disabilities:

1. Should individuals with intellectual or developmental disabilities be classified as a MUP?

2. What are the advantages to being classified as a "health disparities target group?"

3. What are the barriers in your practice or hospital organization to providing care to patients with intellectual or developmental disabilities? Which of these barriers can you improve upon to meet the medical needs of this population?

4. How can primary care physicians and advanced practice providers advocate to reduce disparities in preventive services, medical outcomes, and social determinants of health for this population?

CHAPTER 11

PATIENTS DIAGNOSED WITH "MORBID OBESITY"

> ## DR. BONZO'S BUNGLE OF THE MONTH:
> No Credit Where Credit Was Due

In medical school, I was exposed to teaching physicians who delivered care in many different ways. Some of them dressed casually and used humor with patients, others cried with patients and preferred to be called by their first names, while others wore shirts and ties with white coats and maintained a formal relationship with their patients. My classmates and I adopted different elements of all our teaching physicians' styles of practicing medicine, and we also discarded the parts that we did not consider ideal. One of these areas that I personally discarded was attempting to shame or scare patients.

When we learned about the transtheoretical (stages of change) model of health behavior change[1], we were taught that "precontemplative" patients did not have the intention of changing their negative health behaviors in the foreseeable future. After later speaking with actual patients, I saw physicians who became frustrated arguing with these patients to stop smoking, begin exercising, etc. I learned that it is nearly impossible to know what "button to press" to motivate a given patient. I have seen patients frightened enough by a diagnosis of a benign pulmonary (lung) nodule that they quit smoking on that same day, while other patients of mine have continued to smoke despite a diagnosis of lung cancer.

In my post-residency career, I have embraced motivational interviewing techniques to see what medical issues patients would like to prioritize at their visits. If something feels very important to me, I typically just relay my concerns briefly and leave the door open to future discussions. An example of this that I used in the past was, "Quitting smoking is probably the best thing that most people can do for their health, so let me know if you ever want to talk about it in the future." When patients are contemplative about changing their health behaviors, or when they are ready for action, I try to be compassionate and nonjudgmental—although, like everyone else, my own personal biases sometimes lead me to put my foot in my mouth and end up with material for a bungle of the month.

Speaking of which, let us discuss an encounter that I had with a patient diagnosed with so-called "morbid obesity;" she was a young adult woman who weighed close to 300 pounds. She had switched to our clinic as a new patient and was coming in for her first outpatient follow-up of high blood pressure with us. Her hypertension was relatively well-controlled by a single medication, and I ordered routine surveillance labs of her potassium level and kidney function. She did not have any other concerns, so I told her that weight loss was something that I was interested in talking about in the future whenever she was willing. She hung her head a little and said that it was fine to discuss it now, so I began describing the impact that obesity has on high blood pressure.

I told her that, with significant weight loss, she might be able to eventually discontinue her antihypertensive medication. When I said this, a tear rolled down her cheek, which surprised me given that I was using what I thought was gentle and nonjudgmental language. I was curious if my words were harsh or if she was experiencing fear about the impact of obesity on her health.

My patient told me that it was frustrating because she thought she was doing everything she could, but it never seemed to be enough for her doctors; that was one of the reasons that she switched to our office. More tears started to roll as she informed me that she had lost close to one hundred pounds over the past two years, including fifty pounds in the previous twelve months. She was doing a combination of walking and jogging five days a week, with the goal of eventually being able to run for thirty minutes continuously without taking breaks. She ate at least five servings of fruits and vegetables per day, and she rarely had anything to drink except water. As a result, she had already had one of her blood pressure medications discontinued, as she was previously taking two of them.

My bungle was obviously my assumption that she was not living a healthy lifestyle and had not already done the very things that I was going to recommend. You would think I would have learned my lesson from my previous blunders surrounding religion, sexual orientation, and race, but if it was that easy this book would have only had one chapter.

DEFINITIONS

Body mass index (BMI), which is often used as a surrogate for determining a person's healthy weight, is calculated by dividing a person's weight in kilograms (kg) by the square of their height in meters (m^2). For adults a BMI below 18.5 (kg/m^2) is considered underweight, a BMI between 18.5–24.9 is considered normal weight, a BMI between 25–29.9 is considered *overweight,* and a BMI of 30 or higher is diagnostic of *obesity.* Obesity is further subdivided into different categories:[2]

- Class I obesity: BMI 30 to <35
- Class II obesity: BMI 35 to <40
- Class III obesity: BMI 40 or higher

Class III obesity is sometimes referred to as "*severe obesity*," and it was previously known as "*morbid obesity*." To me, the word "morbid" has often invoked an image of something that is disturbing or repulsive, so I have always felt that referring to obesity in this way was unsettling. My teaching physicians in school reassured me that a lot of medical terms seemed offensive but were just part of the bizarre language of medicine, including the term "incompetent" cervix. However, one of my new patients in residency would have sided with me based on a discussion about why she was switching to our clinic.

She obtained a copy of her medical records for some administrative reason that I cannot remember, but she was offended that her previous doctor had referred to her obesity as "morbid." Since then,

I have typically used the patient's BMI as their diagnosis code (i.e., "BMI >40") instead of using the phrase "morbid obesity." Although combating *fatphobia* in healthcare requires systemic change—you knew that was coming—we should still be responsible for our individual language and behavior.

BIAS ASSOCIATED WITH OBESITY

Systemic biases associated with people who have disabilities share some similarities with people diagnosed with obesity, but one common difference is the assignment of blame. No one blames a patient for requiring a wheelchair to ambulate, but obese patients are often blamed for their diagnosis because the idea is that they can lose weight and correct it if they tried hard enough (this should invoke images of my father's tobacco use as described in Chapter 2 and Chapter 9). Aside from patients with untreated hypothyroidism or an endocrine disorder, many cases of obesity are viewed by society as a simple case of taking in more calories than a person uses up. The simple solution in the eyes of many is to either eat fewer calories or exercise more.

Softening of language from "morbid obesity" to "severe obesity," or even the use of the word "obesity" alone is still associated with significant stigma and weight bias according to a review article by Puhl and Brownell.[3] In their review, they found that approximately one in four nurses admitted to being "repulsed" by obese patients; this should not be surprising given my anecdote from Chapter 2 about the OB/GYN who described pelvic examinations on large women as being "unpleasant." Other, non-clinical professionals also harbor stereotypes of obese patients as being lazy, undisciplined, and less competent in their fields. Studies of both clinicians—including physicians, nurses, and even medical students—and employers revealed a view of obese patients as having poor self-control or being mentally weak.[4,5]

HEALTH DISPARITIES AND INEQUITIES ASSOCIATED WITH OBESITY

Although it is based on population-level data, the use of BMI as a proxy for optimal health has its limitations. People with a BMI >30 overall have higher rates of gallbladder disease, type 2 diabetes mellitus, nonalcoholic steatohepatitis ("fatty liver"), gout, colon cancer, and breast cancer[6]. However, at an individual patient care level, BMI does not accurately predict obesity-related complications; it is also a poor predictor of percent of body fat.[7] Studies of the National Football League (NFL) reveal an almost universal presence of overweight and a more than 25 percent prevalence of at least class II obesity, although many NFL players are world class athletes who have a lower percent body fat than most people you will meet in your day-to-day life.[8]

With the specific impact of obesity on an individual patient being uncertain, what is more certain is the bias and stigma that we mentioned previously. Patients with a BMI >30 are more likely to have delayed preventive services and to not achieve the optimal patient experience that we have discussed with the triple aim of healthcare (see Chapter 2 for details).[9,10] In unpublished data from one of my hospital organizations a few years ago, a survey of almost 500 patients described feelings of disrespectful treatment and negative attitudes by providers. We also received complaints about medical equipment being too small and the embarrassment of being weighed in public spaces. I have also heard numerous complaints from patients who receive unsolicited advice to lose weight, which I was guilty of in my bungle of the month described above.

COMBATING FATPHOBIA IN HEALTHCARE

A lot of the techniques and methods that we have discussed so far in this book should be used to combat weight bias in healthcare. This includes perpetual self-assessment and reflection to scan for implicit and explicit bias at the provider level. This book highlights several groups that experience systemic bias, so healthcare organizations should frequently have focused didactic or training sessions to ensure that target groups of interest are being assessed. Clinics, hospitals, and academic health centers should also measure institutional bias, as my affiliated hospital organization did. When patients report embarrassment about having their weight reported verbally in a hallway with other patients standing around, a systemic fix for this would be to move the scale into a private room. That way, if an individual nurse or medical assistant was not aware of the way this made patients feel, it would at least not be within earshot of other patients and staff.

There are undoubtedly times that patients will require a larger blood pressure cuff, speculum, or gown. The nurses that I have worked with try not to yell down the hallway or make loud requests for these items; and when we are forced to request an item out loud from someone else, we have ways to refer to them that are not as fatphobic. Instead of asking for an extra-large speculum, I ask for "the blue speculum," or if I need an extra-large gown, I ask for the "white gown." Drawing inspiration from Zachary Fenell's approach as described in Chapter 10, the table below describes some alternate ways to discuss the care of patients with severe obesity, with the understanding that everyone will not agree about what language is acceptable and what language is not.

POTENTIAL ALTERNATIVE LANGUAGE WHEN DISCUSSING PATIENTS WITH BMI >30	
Commonly Used Term	Potential Replacement Term
Obese	Person/patient of size
Willpower	Commitment
Diet	Eating style
Exercise/exercise program	Activity style/physical activity
Ideal weight	Healthy weight
Good/bad	What works for you

KNOWLEDGE, ATTITUDES, AND SKILLS

Knowledge

- Patients labeled as obese experience significant stigma and weight bias from the general population and from health care professionals, including doctors and nurses.

- Obese patients are often stereotyped as being lazy or lacking in motivation to improve their health.

- Despite having an increased risk of chronic diseases, metabolic disorders, and various types of cancer, people with a BMI >30 are less likely to receive appropriate preventive services.

Attitudes

- As with other target groups described in this book, generalizations made about people with elevated BMI cannot be reliably or consistently applied to members of this population.

- We should consider alternative language that is less stigmatizing, such as substituting "BMI >40" for "morbid obesity" or "severe obesity."

- All patients are not the same, so some will have different preferences for what language they favor. For example, some might call themselves "fat," while others might be offended by this word.

Skills

- Continue to measure institutional bias; in this case, scan for bias among patients with a BMI >30 to overcome fatphobia in healthcare.

- Encourage self-reflection for individual biases among your work and academic community regarding attitudes toward obese patients.

- Avoid weighing patients in public hallways within outpatient clinics.

- Develop a communication system that does not embarrass patients with requests for extra-large items.

- Ensure that extra-large items and medical supplies are readily available in rooms.
- Follow evidence-based guidelines about the care of patients diagnosed with obesity.

HOW TO TEACH ABOUT SEVERE OBESITY

Case-based narratives are always an effective way to teach health equity, as they will blend the topics discussed in this book with traditional medical education or continuing education about medical topics. You are welcome to utilize any cases that I have presented, including the bungle of the month. I have often presented the case at the beginning of this chapter and asked the audience what their biggest concerns are about the patient's health. They have almost universally discussed her weight, so then I ask them what their recommendations would be. I rarely receive questions about what she has tried so far, but instead the audience discusses suggestions on how to lose weight. This easily leads to a discussion that reinforces concepts from several previous chapters, including bias, stereotyping, and cultural humility. This is a good time to examine the importance of treating each patient like an individual.

In Chapter 9, we discussed a case that could be used to teach about the diagnosis and management of hyperosmolar hyperglycemic nonketotic coma while also discussing the social determinants of health and homelessness. Cases about obesity can also be used as an opportunity to review evidence-based guidelines from organizations such as the American Association of Clinical Endocrinologists (AACE) and the American College of Endocrinology (ACE).[11] These guidelines are available to the public for free and they discuss several topics that can augment your discussions:

- Individualization of pharmacotherapy in the treatment of obesity
- Use of bariatric surgery for weight loss and treatment of obesity

- Lifestyle/behavioral interventions for obesity.

The AACE/ACE also have clinical practice guidelines for healthy eating that discuss the prevention and treatment of various conditions.[12] These will help your audience to consider the education that we should provide *all* patients to prevent various metabolic and endocrine disorders, and they will allow you the chance to highlight the pitfalls of only focusing on patients with a certain BMI.

CHAPTER 12

RURAL HEALTH DISPARITIES

By the time I completed residency, I was fortunate to have obtained a wide clinical skillset that allowed me to practice broad-spectrum family medicine. This meant providing prenatal care and delivering babies, providing inpatient medical care as a hospitalist, and performing procedures for patients who did not have access to specialists. The academic medical center that I worked for purchased a small, critical access hospital in a rural town, and a few faculty members from my department chose to provide clinical care in that rural hospital for extra income. This was an ideal situation for me because it allowed me to pay off student loans, save up for a house, and keep up my procedural skills.

In a rural location that did not have an OB/GYN and that only had one surgeon and one pediatrician in the entire county, the physicians and physician assistants in the rural hospital's ED were required to manage a wide range of medical conditions without specialty assistance. At the time, the hospital did not have an ultrasound machine, and the only magnetic resonance imaging (MRI) machine was a mobile one that was available two days a week. Given that most of my shifts were on weekends, I never had the luxury of using this MRI machine. I was required to use the basic diagnostic tools that we learned in medical school instead of relying on modern technology.

In the five years I provided care at this rural hospital, I was probably able to handle 95 percent of the medical problems that entered our doors. There were times that our hospital did not have the capacity to handle a situation that I encountered, and we had to transport those patients to a larger tertiary care center. Unless there was inclement weather, patient transports went relatively smooth, but we would occasionally have patients who did not want to be transferred.

We did not have cardiology services in the county, so patients with heart attacks were routinely offered transport to a hospital where they could receive procedural interventions such as a cardiac catheterization. Some patients would tell me that they were not going to leave their hometown and that I would have to find a way to treat them there. These patients would be offered thrombolytic treatment (often known to the lay public as "clot busters") to help dissolve the blockage that caused the heart attack. There was typically a second-line option that was available for patients who insisted on staying at our rural hospital, but sometimes this backup option made me anxious about potential outcomes.

{Content warning for non-clinicians: explicit details of a medical injury described below}
One such episode that was anxiety-provoking for me occurred during a surprisingly slow Saturday afternoon, when a farmer presented to the ED with an injury to his ear. He had lacerated the pinna—which is the external, visible portion of the ear—after falling and striking

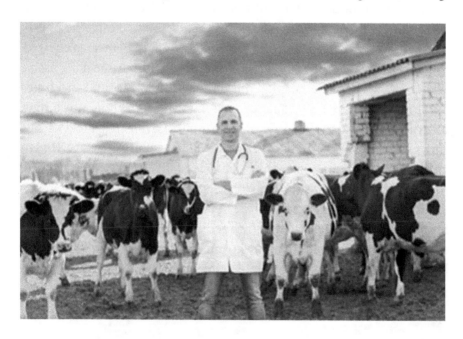

the side of his head on some heavy machinery. The top part of his ear that contains the cartilage had detached from the side of his face, and only the bottom portion with the earlobe was completely intact. After I ruled out an internal brain injury, cleaned the area, checked his hearing, and administered the appropriate pain medication, I told the patient that I needed to transport him to a hospital that had an otolaryngologist (an ear, nose, and throat specialist) available to repair this complex ear laceration. The patient told me, "Oh don't worry about that, Doc! Just sew me up real quick so I can get back to the farm."

I probably spent a good ten minutes telling the patient that I was worried that it would not heal appropriately, but it was to no avail. He was not worried about a poor cosmetic result, so I began to talk about my concerns regarding high infection risk or the possibility of the ear tissue dying and falling off. Since he could hear just fine, he was not worried about going through the remainder of his life with only one full external ear, and he again insisted that I patch him up quickly so that he could get back home.

He finally became increasingly annoyed at my persistence about transferring him forty-five minutes away for his ear repair, and he said that I either needed to start fixing his ear or discharge him home. With that demand, I acquiesced and asked the nurse to prepare a laceration repair tray. While she was doing so, I retreated to my desk in the back of the ED and pulled out a textbook of emergency medicine. I identified the laceration chapter and turned to the section on ears, only to be surprised by a comment about how this type of ear injury was unexpectedly easy to repair. I followed the instructions from the textbook and made my best attempt to suture the top half of his ear back on.

When I finished, the patient thanked me and also remarked, "See, Doc, that wasn't so hard, was it?" I gave him a date to follow-up in the ED for a wound check and suture removal and began to think about that farmer on a daily basis for the next few weeks. I expressed frustration to our medical director about some of the patients in that rural community who were not willing to go to a hospital in another county when they really needed to. I had images of my grandmother who spent her entire life in rural South Carolina and who would refuse to leave town for any reason—although my family was able to convince her to come to my wedding in Georgia.

I stereotyped people living in rural communities as being like my grandmother and being afraid to venture outside of their comfort zone and into larger cities. In the case of this farmer, I was certain that this way of thinking was going to cost him his ear.

A few weeks later, I stopped thinking about the farmer and went on with my daily life, which had become consumed by my first newborn. However, one of my colleagues injected the farmer back into my thoughts during a shift change one evening. After telling the oncoming doctor about the patients remaining in the ED, I was preparing to leave when my colleague said, "Oh my goodness! I've been meaning to talk to you for the past month, but I haven't run into you in a while. Do you remember that guy with the ear laceration that you repaired a month or two ago?" I told him that I did, as my heart began racing and pounding inside my chest.

The other doctor told me that he was the ED physician working the day the farmer returned to have his wound checked and his stitches removed. It probably only took him five to ten seconds to say this, but it felt like an eternity, and the suspense was killing me. The wide mouth and eyes of my coworker were perceived by me to be disgust as I prepared for my peer to tell me that he had been wanting to warn me about how terrible the outcome of the ear repair was. But it was actually the opposite.

The other ED doctor remarked, "That ear repair looked beautiful! How in the world did you learn how to do that?!" As my heart rate and breathing returned to normal, I told him the story of that day, and lamented how that farmer had refused transport. My colleague responded that he was not surprised based on the discussion that he had with that same farmer at the follow-up visit. It turns out that one of his family members was dealing with a serious medical issue which had significant social ramifications for their household. The farmer really needed to get back home to help deal with a problem, which honestly was an issue that one of us from the ED could have driven down the street to help him resolve.

I never took the time to ask the patient why he felt the need to get back home so quickly; I assumed that he was like many of the other rural patients or my grandmother who just did not want to leave their rural community. My patient expressed gratitude that he was able to have his ear repaired right there, and he had a very good medical and cosmetic result. If I had taken the time to just ask him a few questions, our social worker or one of the hospital staff could have helped him to resolve the urgent matter back home, and he probably would not have had a problem with being transferred to the larger hospital.

DEFINITIONS AND DEMOGRAPHICS

Geographic definitions vary depending on which organizational guidelines are utilized; most definitions use county data to determine rural status. The Office of Management and Budget (OMB) defines counties with at least 50,000 people as *metropolitan*, while counties with less than 50,000 people but more than 10,000 people are *micro-politan*; counties with fewer than 10,000 people are classified as "neither," or as "non-metropolitan/non-micropolitan."[1] The OMB specifically uses the term *"rural"* to specify counties that are not part of *a metropolitan statistical area (MSA),* which many analysts interpret as counties with fewer than 50,000 people. Using this definition, rural/non-metropolitan counties contain approximately 15 percent of the United States population (46.2 million people); interestingly, rural counties comprise almost three-fourths (72 percent) of the land mass in this country despite accounting for less than one-sixth of the population.

The U.S. Census Bureau defines geography in binary terms as *urbanized areas* with populations of at least 50,000 people, or as *urban clusters* with less than 50,000 people but more than 2,500 people.[2] Although this is often considered to coincide with the OMB definition, the Census does not technically define rural counties. They define urban regions as being areas that are "densely settled," but their boundaries do not always follow clear city or county boundaries and borders. Areas that are incorporated municipalities or unincorporated cities and towns can all be considered either urban or rural depending on their proximity to densely settled populations. According to the U.S. Census Bureau categorizations, a larger proportion of the country is considered rural compared to the OMB definitions. According to the Census, 19.3 percent of the U.S. population is rural, and rural areas comprise more than 95 percent of the nation's land mass.

The Federal Office of Rural Health Policy (FORHP) utilizes Rural-Urban Commuting Area (RUCA) codes to differentiate between its binary categories of rural and urban. RUCA codes are categorized from one to ten based on decreasing size, population density, and primary commuting flows. Using U.S. Census data, tracts inside metropolitan counties with codes greater than or equal to four (i.e., codes four through ten) are considered *rural*, while most other counties are considered *urban*. There are exceptions, however, as some counties within census tracts with codes two and three that are long distances from critical services are classified as rural. The size of Rural America, based on the FORHP categorization, defines a population that falls in between those described per the OMB and U.S. Census rural definitions. Using the RUCA classification, the FORHP defines 18 percent of the population as rural, and rural counties encompass 84 percent of the U.S. land mass.

In addition to the federal agencies described above, there are other definitions for rural, urban, and suburban communities or counties. In general, using the definition of a county with a population of fewer than 50,000 people will encompass the majority of rural areas as defined by most organizations. Overall, the designation of rural is important in discussing healthcare and health equity because these communities tend to have higher rates of poverty and, by definition, they have smaller populations.

Higher rates of poverty (Image 25) in rural areas are unsurprisingly linked to lower rates of healthcare coverage and inability to afford medications or medical interventions. Fewer people bring fewer health care employees and physicians, and geographic isolation of some rural communities can impede access to medical specialties. For communities that are particularly small and secluded, the term *"frontier"* is often used to specify rural areas with a population density ≤6 persons per square mile.[3] Past definitions of frontier also required a travel distance of at least sixty minutes to a medical facility that could perform a cesarean delivery ("C-section") or provide advanced cardiac life support (ACLS – management of cardiac arrest).

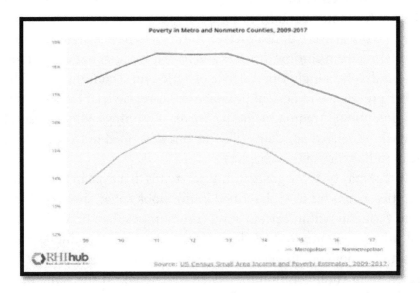

As we discuss rural counties, it is important to remember that county lines are not drawn in a consistent or uniform manner, as they were historically influenced by geographic landmarks (e.g., rivers, state borders) or by the distribution of certain populations. As a result, there is a wide variation in the amount of land or square footage that constitutes each county. In addition to being unequal in size, proximity to MSAs has a significant influence on the experience of people in rural areas.

For example, a county could have 25,000 people but it could be located next to a county that contains hundreds of thousands of people and has a large academic medical center. Conversely, a different county could have 45,000 people while being surrounded by all rural counties and lacking a major tertiary care medical center. In those scenarios, the smaller rural county might have access to a much wider range of healthcare services than the larger rural county. As with the other target groups that we have discussed so far, rural communities are not identical and have a significant level of heterogeneity.

RURAL HEALTH DISPARITIES AEND INEQUITIES

In our introduction to health disparities in Chapter 1, we discussed a lack of technological infrastructure in many rural areas that carries over into the delivery of healthcare.[4] Rural areas have a higher burden of suffering from chronic diseases and have less access to healthy food options despite a higher prevalence of agricultural communities. The higher prevalence of agricultural laborers can also lead to high rates of unintentional trauma including burns, poisonings, and industrial or machine-related accidents (like the one described in my bungle of the month earlier in this chapter).

There may be some general cultural trends that exist in rural communities, but as we have described in this book so far, there could be more variation within certain rural communities than between rural and urban communities. We have discouraged stereotyping and assumptions about our target groups, so we will encourage treating each person from rural communities as an individual. At the same time, we should be aware of unequal health outcomes that are prevalent among the groups that we are discussing, so let us explore some of these trends in rural areas.

People living in rural communities are more likely to report being in poor health, yet they are also more likely to delay medical care due to cost.[5] Data from the Behavioral Risk Factor Surveillance System (BRFSS) reveals that worsened health in rural communities is related more to poverty, unemployment, and higher rates of obesity, than it is to county population size.[6] People living in rural or non-metropolitan counties have higher rates of smoking and moderate alcohol use, and they are less likely to meet the physical activity and exercise recommendations of 150 minutes per week.[7]

In Chapter 11, we discussed the correlation between elevated BMI and worsening health, not only because of a trend towards higher rates of chronic disease and cancer, but also because of stigma from health care providers and unequal provision of preventive services.[8] Therefore, it is not surprising that rural counties, which have higher obesity rates, have multiple factors that influence health outcomes in those areas.

Residents of rural counties have a lower life expectancy compared to people living in non-rural counties, and as the life expectancy has overall improved for both rural and urban areas since the turn of the millennium, the gap between them has not changed.[9] During the brief, temporary periods of time when the gap has narrowed, it is typically related to worsening in urban areas, not to improvements in rural counties. A similar trend exists for infant mortality (Image 26), which has gradually improved nationwide over the past few decades while the gap between metropolitan and non-metropolitan infant mortality has actually increased in size. Even for conditions that are less frequent in rural areas, some of them still have higher associated death rates, as demonstrated by data from the CDC, National Vital Statistics System, National Cancer Institute, and National Program of Cancer Registries.

Although rural areas have a lower overall incidence of cancer, they have higher death rates from cancer compared to urban areas. In one analysis of a decade's worth of data, the annual age-adjusted death rates for cancer decreased in the United States, but the rate of decrease was slower in non-metropolitan areas, which further widened the gap between rural and urban cancer mortality.[10]

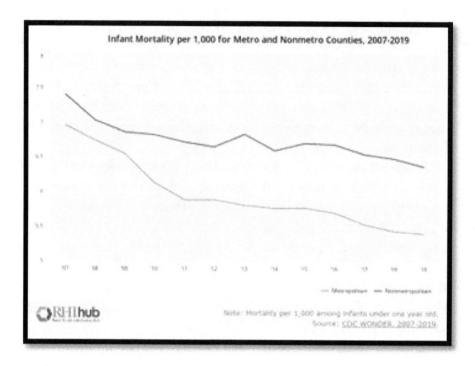

Infant Mortality per 1,000 for Metro and Nonmetro Counties, 2007-2019

The rural South has particularly high rates of cardiovascular risk factors, which is concerning given that heart disease is the leading cause of death in the United States, and stroke is the third- and fifth-leading cause of death for females and males, respectively (Image 27).[11] Cancer is the second leading cause of death for all genders and sexes, and the previous paragraph outlined the disparities in cancer mortality that exist in rural areas. The result is that the major causes of death in this country are either more prevalent or more deadly for people living in rural counties. Previously described health behaviors such as increased smoking and decreased physical activity all contribute to the development of acute and chronic diseases in rural areas, but systemic barriers to accessing healthcare in a timely manner may increase the death rate from these conditions as well.

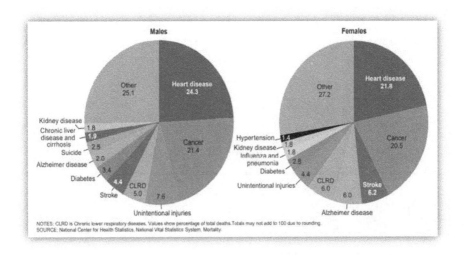

Males   Females

NOTES: CLRD is Chronic lower respiratory diseases. Values show percentage of total deaths. Totals may not add to 100 due to rounding.
SOURCE: National Center for Health Statistics, National Vital Statistics System, Mortality.

I attended medical school in Georgia and my family medicine residency was in North Carolina. I often heard my teaching physicians say that we were in the "Stroke Belt" of the United States. Looking at data from the CDC and Rural Health Information Hub on death rates from stroke (Image 28), you might conclude that it is not surprising that states in the Southern United States are referred to as such; the results are similar for death rates from heart disease.

At the same time, we have discussed that "words matter," and in recent years I have become concerned about the possible stigmatizing nature of language like "Stroke Belt," as it has the potential to cause us to view the health disparities of the rural South as an inevitability. It also could lead to some of us viewing rural Southerners as biologically or socially flawed, depending on if the point of view is on the medical outcomes or on the potential health behaviors that increase the risk of some of these diseases.

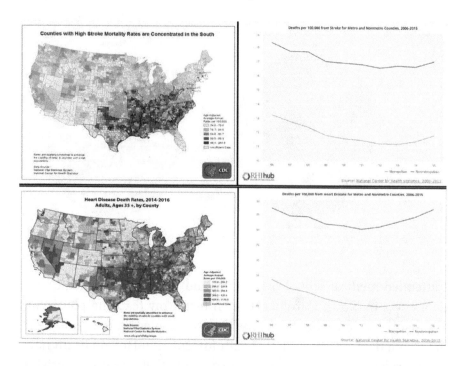

A phenomenon with the potential to exacerbate the inequities described above is the closing of rural hospitals in areas that already have physician shortages. Rural counties have difficulty recruiting and retaining physicians, so closing the places where rural physicians work can negatively impact community health. Per a recent report from the Physician Workforce in my home state of Georgia, there are eight counties that do not have a single physician, and several more that do not have a primary care physician; eleven counties do not have a family physician, thirty-seven counties are without an internal medicine physician, and sixty-three counties lack a pediatrician.[12] Approximately half of the counties in Georgia do not have an OB/GYN, and more than half do not have a psychiatrist. Almost all of these counties with physician shortages are rural counties.

In the past twelve years, nine rural hospitals have closed in Georgia, mostly due to financial reasons.[13] When I have given visiting lectures on this topic, I often scan the data in the states where I will be presenting to see if they experience similar obstacles in rural locales. Via this process, I recently learned that eighteen of Michigan's seventy-one rural hospitals were reported as having a high risk of closing according to Guidehouse—formerly known as Navigant—a Chicago-based national healthcare consulting firm (Image 29).[14] In addition to Georgia and Michigan, other states determined to have a high financial risk to their rural hospitals include Minnesota, Maine, Alaska, Alabama, Mississippi, Iowa, Oklahoma, Kansas, Arkansas, and Kentucky. Although North Carolina was not included in this list, a separate report from the North Carolina Rural Health Research Program detailed the closing of nineteen rural hospitals. Since January 2010, at least 134 rural hospitals nationwide have been forced to close.[15]

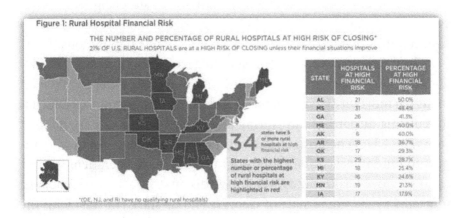

Figure 1: Rural Hospital Financial Risk

THE NUMBER AND PERCENTAGE OF RURAL HOSPITALS AT HIGH RISK OF CLOSING*
21% OF U.S. RURAL HOSPITALS are at a HIGH RISK OF CLOSING unless their financial situations improve

STATE	HOSPITALS AT HIGH FINANCIAL RISK	PERCENTAGE AT HIGH FINANCIAL RISK
AL	21	50.0%
MS	31	48.4%
GA	26	41.3%
ME	8	40.0%
AK	6	40.0%
AR	18	36.7%
OK	17	29.3%
KS	29	28.7%
MI	18	25.4%
KY	16	24.6%
MN	19	21.3%
IA	17	17.9%

34 states have 5 or more rural hospitals at high financial risk

States with the highest number or percentage of rural hospitals at high financial risk are highlighted in red

*(DE, NJ, and RI have no qualifying rural hospitals)

COMBATING SYSTEMIC BIAS IN RURAL HEALTHCARE

As we scan for health disparities, we have encouraged an intersectional view of the various target groups in this book; this also applies to people living in rural areas. For example, we highlighted that infant mortality rates are higher in rural counties, but they are especially worse in the counties with high poverty rates.[16] This is particularly driven by higher rates of sudden unexpected death in infancy (SUDI—frequently known as sudden infant death syndrome, or SIDS), so interventions to improve infant mortality—such as community education programs about safe sleeping positions—may focus initially on high-poverty areas. After our discussions from Chapter 9, it should not be surprising that the social determinants of health play a major role in infant survival. According to a retrospective cohort study by Ehrenthal et al., socioeconomic disadvantages are the largest contributors to infant mortality in rural counties, more so than limitations in healthcare access or increased hazardous health behaviors.[17]

Aside from income level, the distribution of other demographics in rural areas are associated with varying medical outcomes. Rural counties overall have had a lower prevalence rate of COVID-19, but counties that have higher rates of obesity and smoking have had a higher prevalence rate.[18] Rural counties with larger populations of young adults and/or Black people have had higher rates and more rapid spread of SARS-CoV-2. In addition to infant mortality and infectious diseases, rural counties have a large burden of suffering from other causes of premature death, and this disparity is more pronounced in communities that have larger Black or Indigenous populations.[19]

The CDC offers several strategies to decrease the excess morbidity and mortality associated with chronic diseases in rural areas.[20] As with maternal mortality (see Chapter 3) and the other systemic approaches to reducing disparities, measuring and reporting data is a crucial first step. The CDC encourages states to provide adequate financial support to fund interventions and programs that have been demonstrated to improve health outcomes. I have discussed the dismal maternal mortality in my home state of Georgia and its stark contrast with the improvement in maternal mortality seen in California in recent years. Using the CDC approach, other states should fund the same types of data reporting, protocol implementation, and educational initiatives that worked in California.

The CDC also recommends promoting health and healthcare delivery through the use of digital formats such as *"telemedicine"* or *"telehealth."* Telehealth interventions have been demonstrated to be a feasible intervention for rural areas that have difficulty recruiting and retaining physicians, and telehealth is associated with decreased healthcare costs and increased patient satisfaction in rural communities (this should sound familiar from our "triple aim" discussions in Chapter 2 and Chapter 11).[21] Lack of broadband internet services might not seem like a healthcare problem, but a reliable internet connection with video streaming capabilities is necessary for effective telemedicine.

Over the past decade, increases in insurance coverage in rural areas were mostly related to the expansion of Medicaid and enrollment in the Health Insurance Marketplace that occurred under the Affordable Care Act (ACA). In one analysis, insurance status for rural veterans was three times higher in states that expanded Medicaid under the ACA, and low-income veterans in particular saw a decline in the number of them that were uninsured.[22] Veterans living in rural areas are more likely to live in the South, and they also have a high prevalence of markers of poor economic well-being including uninsured status. We have already discussed in Chapter 1 and Chapter 10 that veterans are a target group with higher rates of disability, so lacking access to healthcare because of insurance status compounds the health challenges seen in rural areas for this patient population.

The purpose of this book is not to assess the financial or political pros and cons of the ACA, but rather to highlight that universal healthcare coverage does decrease health disparities for vulnerable populations. If the ACA is not going to be the path forward, then policymakers and legislators should propose alternatives to ensure that the poor, our veterans, and people living in rural communities can access high-quality medical care.

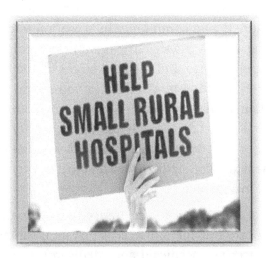

A critique of the fee-for-service system of healthcare in the United States and the poor reimbursement for uninsured or publicly insured patients are not just discussions for policy experts. As a society, we must figure out a way to make rural hospitals more financially solvent if we want to achieve health equity for rural and underserved populations. The American Hospital Association Rural Report identified seven specific challenges that threaten the survival of rural hospitals:[23]

1. Low volume
2. Challenging payer mix
3. Challenging patient mix
4. Geographic isolation
5. Workforce shortages
6. Limited access to essential services
7. Aging infrastructure and access to capital.

In response to the Rural Report, here are some parting thoughts to consider if we want to achieve health equity in rural communities:

1. Health care providers and hospital systems currently receive more money for seeing more patients and for performing more procedures. A cardiac catheterization procedure is valued more than a community intervention to decrease cardiovascular risk. A physician is reimbursed more for living in a metropolitan area and seeing a large volume of patients than they are for living in a rural area and seeing a lower volume of patients. Our lawmakers should provide financial support for rural hospitals and provide incentives for physicians and advanced practice providers to work in rural areas. Loan repayment and competitive salaries are just a couple of these potential incentives.

2. Our current system for insurance reimbursement encourages health care providers to accept private insurance over public insurance (i.e., Medicaid and Medicare). I have lived in two

cities where a large percentage of specialists do not accept Medicaid. Patients living in rural counties are viewed as being covered by a "challenging payer mix" because of one of the major problems with our system—it is not financially beneficial for private practices to accept Medicaid, Medicare, or the Marketplace insurances. I have heard many physicians challenge me on why they should accept Medicaid when it pays only $0.40 for every dollar that a private company reimburses while doing the same amount of work. Our government must be bold enough to provide equal reimbursement for public insurance, knowing that a healthy public will help to recoup those costs down the road (see Chapter 9 if you have any doubts).

3. This chapter has clearly outlined the "challenging patients" that the American Hospital Association is referencing. Practicing medicine is challenging, and as a specialty we never back down from any biomedical challenge. Surgeons can transplant organs into other people, perform brain surgery, and operate on a fetus while they are still *in utero*. Surely, we can learn how to address the social determinants of health in a more effective manner. As above in #1, we must provide better reimbursement for health care providers who address the social challenges that patients and clients experience, especially since we know that this process would improve morbidity and mortality to a greater extent than traditional clinical care.

4. The geographic isolation of rural communities demonstrates how critical it is for governments to provide fiscal support so that rural hospitals can remain open. Also, the solutions discussed in #1 above will increase the number of physicians who practice in rural areas. Continuing education, shared practices, and telehealth consultation can also help rural clinicians provide high-quality, evidence-based care that is known to decrease inequities.

5. One major contributor to workforce shortages is that it takes several years of postbaccalaureate education to become a

physician, physician assistant, nurse, nurse practitioner, physical therapist, etc. When a rural community loses one of these health care professionals, their only choice is to recruit another, as it takes so long for someone to complete the requisite training for a "homegrown" replacement. Many health professions schools are recruiting students from rural areas, as they are more likely to return to their hometown or other rural communities to practice; they are also more likely to stay long term.

6. I described my experience of the divide between medicine and public health in Chapter 9, and I also explained how social factors contribute to health outcomes. The 10 Essential Public Health Services as described by the CDC (Image 30) highlights how policymakers, legislators, public health workers, and the healthcare workforce can come together to promote community health.

7. We have discussed how improvements in broadband internet access can increase the potential for effective rural telehealth opportunities. Also, improvements in infrastructure can support the social determinants of health that we have discussed at length.

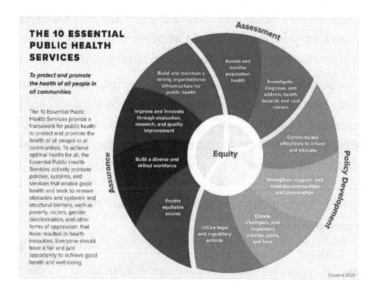

KNOWLEDGE, ATTITUDES, AND SKILLS

Knowledge

- Rural communities have a higher burden of suffering from chronic diseases, and residents of rural counties are more likely to rate themselves as being in poor health.

- Rural residents have a higher prevalence of health behaviors associated with worse health outcomes (e.g., smoking, sedentary lifestyle).

- People living in rural areas are more likely to live in poverty and have limitations on their access to high-quality healthcare.

- Many of the health disparities seen in rural communities are associated with structural inequities in employment, poverty, and educational attainment.

- Telehealth programs have high rates of patient and provider satisfaction and are associated with lower healthcare costs.

Attitudes

- It is important to consider the intersection of rural status and other demographic factors—race, disability status, obesity, etc.—in attempting to reduce rural health disparities.

- Rural communities are very diverse, and there is even significant diversity within specific rural counties; for example, the burden of suffering from various diseases varies within a county based on age, gender, and other factors.

- Addressing social determinants of health such as poverty and education level is a critical piece in eliminating health inequities in rural communities.

- Because of the access barriers that they experience, lack of health insurance is a problem that can be even worse for residents of rural counties compared to urban or suburban areas.

- Broad-spectrum primary care physicians should be valued, as their presence has been correlated with an improvement in morbidity and mortality across the country.

Skills

- Use advocacy to encourage policymakers and legislators to incentivize practice in rural areas for physicians and advanced practice providers.

- Provide financial, organizational, and consultant support for obstetric care provided by family physicians and midwives, particularly in areas that have a shortage of obstetricians.

- Utilize interventions and programs that are evidence-based and have been shown to improve outcomes in other areas around the country.

- Increase the availability of broadband internet services in rural counties so that telehealth interventions can be implemented and consistently utilized.

HOW TO TEACH ABOUT RURAL HEALTH DISPARITIES

Many of the themes from previous chapters are critical in understanding rural health inequities, so my advice on teaching about rural health issues will depend on whether or not you have reviewed the previous chapters—especially Chapter 9—with your audience. If you have discussed the social determinants of health in a previous session, then you can begin to explore other common challenges in rural counties; if not, then I would recommend doing so either in conjunction with the rural health session or at a prior date. The population-based model of patient-centered care from the Medical College of Wisconsin (Image 31) can be used as a template to discuss the various domains that contribute to the health of communities. Depending on your audience or area of focus, you can investigate public policy or organizational changes that could overcome various barriers in those domains if you were located in a rural setting.

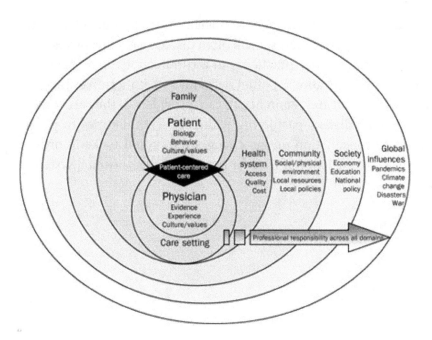

We have repeatedly discussed the importance of *measuring systemic and institutional bias*, so this is always one of the major points of discussion for any of the target groups. I have discovered that audiences are more engaged when the conversations include topics they are interested in, so a good pre-session activity is to have participants explore rural health disparities within their field. For example, they can look up (and share with the group on a volunteer basis) which rural health disparities exist for their current or desired specialty, and they can begin to discuss population-level interventions that could reduce these disparities. (If they do not have a specialty yet, they can describe which inequities they believe have the highest burden of suffering.)

For example, if someone is interested in general surgery and learns that a rural community has high rates of trauma, they could share this information with the group and discuss how they would address the problem. This could lead to discussions on how one might implement a Stop the Bleed (STB) program, for example.[24]

Access to high-quality healthcare is where I typically end, and the point of view depends on the audience that I am addressing. In didactic sessions with resident physicians, medical students, or other health professions students, I will often discuss what incentives would lead them to consider practicing in a rural county. In sessions with healthcare organizations, I often delve into what incentives they have offered to recruit and retain health care providers. If they are in urban areas, then I discuss partnering with rural communities to provide telehealth consultation or any changes they could make in order to enhance the efficiency of transfer services to their hospital system.

CHAPTER 13

HARM REDUCTION AND PEOPLE WHO USE DRUGS

BACKGROUND

Do not worry, there *will* be a bungle of the month for this chapter; I just need to give some background and context first, so allow me to go a little out of order. In Chapter 6, we discussed my work as the PI on a FOCUS grant that funded a large-scale HIV and HCV screening program in non-traditional settings such as the ED. We developed our screening protocols based on the recommendations of some of the major public health and disease prevention organizations in the United States. The CDC, American Association for the Study of Liver Diseases (AASLD), and Infectious Diseases Society of America (IDSA) recommend screening individuals aged eighteen years and older at least once for HCV,[1,2] while the USPSTF recommends HCV testing for adults aged eighteen to seventy-nine.[3,4] These organizations also recommend testing patients at increased risk of HCV infection, including incarcerated individuals and people who inject drugs. (More on this in a moment.)

The USPSTF recommends screening for HIV among adults and adolescents aged fifteen to sixty-five years, for all pregnant women (which is generally agreed upon to be any pregnant person), and for people below age fifteen or above age sixty-five who are at increased risk of infection.[5] The CDC recommends routine HIV screening for all people aged thirteen to sixty-four, especially in settings that have a disease prevalence of at least 0.1 percent.[6] The CDC recommends opt-out testing, in which testing is performed on all eligible people unless they decline, regardless of their perceived risk. This routine opt-out screening is intended to increase screening rates and decrease the stigma linked to HIV testing. It also removes the potential for health care providers to inaccurately stereotype patients as needing or not needing an HIV test; hopefully, by this point of the book, you understand that all of us have the potential to do exactly that without the proper failsafe.

One major benefit of screening and early detection of HIV is that it allows for early treatment with ART, which has been shown to decrease individual AIDS-related mortality, to decrease vertical transmission (i.e., spread from mother to infant during childbirth), and to decrease community viral loads. Early diagnosis of HCV is also related to improved outcomes based on the ability to initiate direct acting antiviral (DAA) medications. DAA therapy has the benefits of inducing a sustained virologic response (i.e., undetectable viral load and essentially a virologic cure) and inducing remission in HCV-related Hodgkin's lymphoma;[7] a recent cohort study also showed decreased mortality in patients treated for chronic HCV infection regardless of whether they had cirrhosis or not.[8]

I previously mentioned that our initial goal was to screen large groups of the population for HIV and HCV, and then to rapidly link patients who test positive to community partners for the initiation of treatment. We also began studying patients who tested negative but had significant risks for acquiring HIV and HCV infection. This revealed a community need for increased access to PrEP services for HIV prevention (again, see Chapter 6), but it also revealed a need for preventive services related to HCV infection.

Risk factors for acquiring HIV infection include condomless sex, vertical transmission, and receiving blood transfusions prior to 1985. Sources of HCV infection include receiving blood transfusions or organ transplants prior to 1992, receiving unregulated tattoos or piercings, and several less-common causes—vertical transmission (6 percent), needle stick injuries, sexual contact, and possibly sharing of household items such as razors.[9] *One major risk factor for both of these viral infections is sharing needles and syringes*, especially for HCV, which can survive outside of the human body for up to three weeks.

Image 11 (Chapter 6) outlined that my home state of Georgia has the highest incidence rate of HIV in the United States, but the Southern region of the country in general has been disproportionately affected by HIV and AIDS. Nearly half (47 percent) of AIDS-related deaths are in the South, even though only 38 percent of the population lives there; the South also accounts for 52 percent of new HIV diagnoses and 53 percent of new AIDS diagnoses.[10] A multistep analysis using cases of acute HCV infection estimated that more than two-thirds of counties vulnerable to HCV outbreaks related to *injection drug use* were located in the South.[11]

In the same way that I aspired to increase access to PrEP in my community, I began to explore ways to decrease the risk of HIV and HCV infection related to the sharing of needles and syringes. Similar to the lack of PrEP services in our county, we discovered that several patients did not have access to DAA therapy for chronic HCV infection; specifically, most of the specialists in our town would not see patients diagnosed with HCV if they had Medicaid or if they lacked health insurance. We developed a training program for our internal medicine and family medicine residency clinics and began to provide DAA treatment for Medicaid patients at these locations. In addition, my FQHC was able to set up a similar program for uninsured patients.[12] However, we did not have any local programs that provided clean needles and syringes for people who inject opioids and other drugs.

A systematic review and meta-analysis of needle and syringe programs (NSPs) revealed a strong association with reduced HIV transmission among people who inject drugs (PWID); they can also help to decrease the transmission of HCV by as much as 50 percent within this population.[13,14] NSPs are also cost effective, as the CDC reports the lifetime cost of treating just one patient with HIV is more than $400,000. Even large NSPs can typically operate on a budget of less than $100,000 annually, and the return on investment is estimated to be $7.58 for every $1 spent.[15]

Although some critics have had concerns that these programs will encourage drug use or create a false sense of security, people who participate in NSPs had a reduction in injection frequency and were more likely to enter and remain in drug treatment.[16] NSPs were legalized in my home state in 2019 after experiencing widespread bipartisan support; Georgia House Bill 217 passed the House by a margin of 166–3 (98 percent in favor) and it passed the Senate by a margin of 45–4 (92 percent in favor).[17]

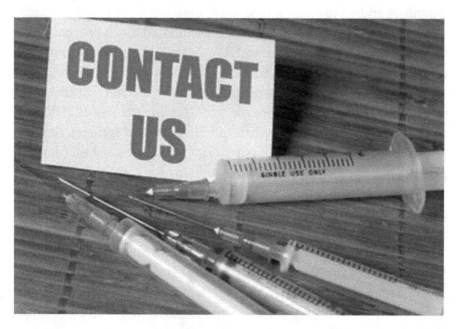

DR. BONZO'S BUNGLE OF THE MONTH:
Just Say No?

The more I researched NSPs, the more convinced I became that they should be the standard of care for precontemplative PWID (see Chapter 2 and Chapter 11 for brief discussions of precontemplation and the transtheoretical stages of change model). I was already convinced that a harm reduction model was the appropriate way to approach healthcare and public health, so this was yet another step in validating this attitude (keep reading for more on harm reduction). I began looking for grants to begin a NSP program, and I was fortunate to make the acquaintance of a fantastic community partner through the No More O.D.s program (https://www.nomore-overdoses.com). I began talking about the importance of using clean needles, syringes, and injection supplies for PWID, and I incorporated information about NSPs into my lectures for our medical students and resident physicians.

While awaiting the development of a formal NSP, one of my residents brought up the idea of temporary fixes for the problem of infectious disease transmission related to injection drug use. I was precepting in the outpatient setting on that day, and the resident had a patient who regularly injected heroin; the resident was discussing the risks of intravenous (IV) drug use with them, but the patient knew that they were not ready to quit using at that time. However, they were interested in infection risk reduction, and the resident had informed them that they could clean their own needles and syringes with bleach and water until we had an established NSP.

I informed the resident that my lectures discussing the "2 x 2 x 2 method" that was studied by the WHO—two flushes with sterile water, two flushes with bleach, and two more flushes with water—did kill more than 95 percent of the HIV virus present in used needles and syringes, but that it was only recommended as a second-line option compared to NSPs.[18,19] One main reason is that people outside of research studies often do not follow the sterilizing technique protocol appropriately, or if they are heavily under the influence of a substance, they may be unable to follow the directions properly. My resident still asked me to discuss this with the patient when I went in to do the evaluation required for teaching physicians who are supervising residents.

When I entered the patient's room, I realized I had stereotyped them in a similar way to how I did with the houseless man in Chapter 9's bungle of the month. I have known several people who have used drugs recreationally and it did not affect their daily life, so I did not have stereotypical images of them. However, after my resident's presentation, I created a stereotype in my mind when I heard about someone using heroin without being able to stop; I am embarrassed to say that I had one image of a recreational drug user versus another image for a "heroin addict." I did not expect to find a married individual—with gainful employment—who mostly used heroin with their spouse but did occasionally run out of injection supplies. These are the times that they borrowed from other people, and they were concerned about their risk of acquiring HIV and HCV infection.

When I explained the "2 x 2 x 2 method," they asked us to either give them a printout or write down the information so that they would remember. They told me that their plan was to collect and pre-clean several syringes ahead of time so that they would have an ample supply. The patient also accepted a prescription for PrEP by the end of the visit, and they said they would get the spouse to make a follow-up appointment for PrEP as well. I had always heard of a definition of addiction that included a significant interference with and negative effects upon daily life caused by drugs. I now realize that those negative effects are not always defined by others in the same way that I define them, and that many people are highly functional and indistinguishable from anyone else in society even when they have high levels of physical dependence on substances such as opioids.

ADDICTION AND HARM REDUCTION

The American Society of Addiction Medicine (ASAM) defines *addiction* as "a treatable, chronic medical disease involving complex interactions among brain circuits, genetics, the environment, and an individual's life experiences."[20] They go on to say that "people with addiction use substances or engage in behaviors that become compulsive and often continue despite harmful consequences." A systematic literature review of definitions of addiction (Sussman and Sussman, 2011) revealed several common elements: suffering negative consequences, loss of control, temporary satiation, and preoccupation with the behavior (or "spilling over" into other aspects of daily life).[21] This review also included a common theme of a desire to shift the subjective experience of self ("appetitive effect"); it also differentiates addiction from compulsion, as compulsions tend to be more spontaneous while addictions involve planning as part of a cyclic pattern of behavior.

In the 1980s and 1990s, a new model of care developed internationally that was an alternative to an idealistic view of medicine in which patients and clients are persuaded to avoid all high-risk behavior.

Instead of a "zero tolerance" policy for risky behavior, scholars such as Eric Single at the University of Toronto demonstrated that more practical goals could reduce adverse outcomes for drug use.[22,23] A *harm reduction* approach attempts to reduce the negative consequences of a behavior as opposed to trying to change or eliminate the behavior. Harm reduction is often linked to the field of addiction medicine, but it can also apply to other health behaviors such as condomless sex. Preventing the acquisition of viral and bacterial infections related to injection drug use was discussed earlier in this chapter, but the prevention of overdose is another aspect of harm reduction.

Harm reduction does not encourage or accelerate the behavior that creates the health risks. NSPs and the prescribing of PrEP do not encourage injection drug use among people who otherwise would not have; similarly, distributing condoms or contraception does not increase sexual activity among adolescents.

ACHIEVING HEALTH EQUITY AND OVERCOMING BARRIERS FOR PEOPLE WHO USE DRUGS

All of the behaviors and obstacles that affect the other target groups discussed in this book also apply to people who use drugs (PWUD). Implicit bias, explicit bias, stereotyping, and prejudicial views of PWUD all contribute to the stigma associated with drug use, which can in turn encourage people to avoid clinical settings. Hopefully, by this stage of the book, you have either developed or refined your skills in how to minimize behaviors that contribute to this stigma.

There are also structural issues that preserve systemic biases for this population, and we have discussed how systemic bias can be more damaging than individual bias. Over two-thirds of the more than 70,000 annual drug overdose deaths in the United States are related to opioid use, including both prescribed and illicit opioids. Medications for addiction treatment (MAT, formerly known as "medication-assisted treatment") such as buprenorphine, methadone, naloxone, and naltrexone can increase abstinence and decrease the risk of overdose and death;[24] however, only one-third of patients treated for opioid use disorder (OUD) receive these treatments with the strongest evidence of efficacy.

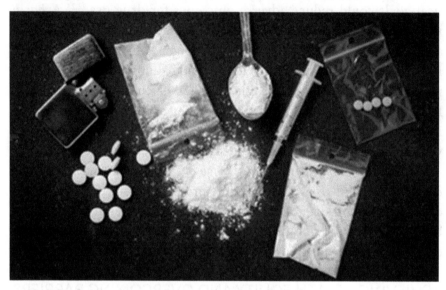

Despite the need for MAT, there are structural barriers that discourage health care providers from regularly prescribing these potentially life-saving therapies. Prescribing methadone for OUD is accompanied by strict federal regulations that typically require daily travel to treatment facilities to obtain the medication. At the time of publication, permission to prescribe buprenorphine requires a waiver that can only be obtained after completing eight hours of training, and only physicians were eligible for this training up until the year 2017. At the time that nurse practitioners and physician assistants were first allowed to obtain buprenorphine waivers, one study revealed that more than half of rural counties did not have a single clinician prescribing this form of MAT.[25]

Although 50 percent of PWID live outside of urban areas, only 30 percent of NSPs are located outside of urban cities. Per current regulations, each health care provider can only prescribe buprenorphine to one hundred patients for the first year after obtaining the waiver, and then the clinician can request to increase their patient limit to 275 patients. As a result, physicians in both urban and rural areas are often not accepting new patients for MAT, and rural counties in particular lack access to NSPs.[26]

In addition to the prescribing of medications for OUD, other clinical practices to decrease the potential complications of drug use are sometimes encountered with systemic barriers. When we attempted to implement age-based opt-out testing for HIV and HCV—as per the aforementioned consensus guidelines—we were met by resistance from some administrators. Some members of the hospital's team wanted to continue with a separate consent form for HIV testing, despite the fact that the CDC had been discouraging separate consents for the previous decade. There was a fear of offending patients by offering them a test for HIV, and one administrator expressed concern that an HIV diagnosis would induce suicidal behavior.

Fortunately, we were able to overcome these impediments by engaging members of our hospital leadership who had medical, clinical, or public health backgrounds. We also involved the information technology (IT) team to configure an electronic medical record (EMR) system to ease the physician workflow in the ED; they accomplished this by automating the process of ordering HIV tests, whereby the EMR scans the patient's chart to see if they are eligible for the test and subsequently recommends that the physician order the test with a simple click on the computer. This resulted in the ED doctors and nurses also becoming vocal supporters of our work.

The idea of elderly patients becoming angry at us for considering the idea that they could be infected with HIV was unfounded, as more than 90 percent of patients who had blood collected in the ED accepted the opt-out testing. Also, the age distribution of positive HIV test results was rather uniform (Image 32).

Even after we allayed the fears of the few concerned administrators regarding HIV screening, we encountered stigma associated with our plans for HCV screening in the outpatient setting. When we expressed a desire to initiate a concerted effort to provide DAA for the treatment of chronic HCV infection, we again encountered some administrative personnel who linked HCV to PWID. One vocal individual asserted that we have to be careful in attracting "that kind of population" to our clinics. When challenging them on this point of view, they could not tell me which hospital system in town was better suited for "those kinds of patients." I also reminded them that we do not approach any other diseases or disorders in that manner.

We were eventually able to convince them to acquiesce on this point as well, but unfortunately, we had to resort to playing off of the same stereotyping that was hindering our administrators from supporting this initiative. We discussed the high rates of HCV infection among the Baby Boomer cohort (i.e., people born between 1945–1965), and the image of grandmothers who had chronic HCV infection from short-term drug use during Woodstock made them ultimately welcome our DAA clinic plans.

KNOWLEDGE, ATTITUDES, AND SKILLS

Knowledge

- Harm reduction focuses on minimizing negative consequences of a behavior instead of trying to eliminate the behavior, especially if a patient is not ready to change that behavior.

- Current guidelines recommend age-based screening for blood-borne viral infections, such as HIV and HCV.

- Early diagnosis and initiation of antiviral medication decreases morbidity and mortality associated with HIV and HCV, and it also decreases community viral loads and spread of these infections.

- Providing clean needles and syringes to people who inject drugs decreases HIV and HCV transmission.

Attitudes

- Harm reduction does not influence people to increase high-risk behavior.

- Needle and syringe programs will not encourage drug use, but they will paradoxically decrease drug use and increase entrance into rehabilitation programs.

- Screening for bloodborne viral infections by age increases diagnoses and decreases the chance that stereotyping will influence the decision to order these tests.

- Interdisciplinary collaboration is critical when implementing population-level screening programs that benefit PWID; be ready for barriers.

- Approaches to achieve health equity for PWUD should be patient-centered and community-partnered, and they should utilize a harm reduction model.

Skills

- Encourage, support, and incentivize advanced practice providers (e.g., physician assistants, nurse practitioners) to obtain buprenorphine waivers or training in other methods of MAT.

    Some medical schools are even including buprenorphine waiver training into the graduate medical education curriculum.

- Use age-based guidelines to screen for viral infections associated with intravenous drug use, as they are more effective in detecting HIV and HCV compared to clinical gestalt or risk factor-based screening.

- Use an opt-out testing strategy for HIV and HCV screening.

- In addition to distribution of safer injection supplies, NSPs should also provide the following:

    1. substance abuse and harm reduction counseling

    2. referrals for substance abuse disorder treatment

    3. training and provision of naloxone to reverse opioid overdose

    4. referrals and linkage to care for prevention or treatment of sexually transmitted and bloodborne infections, and screening for HIV, viral hepatitis, and STIs.

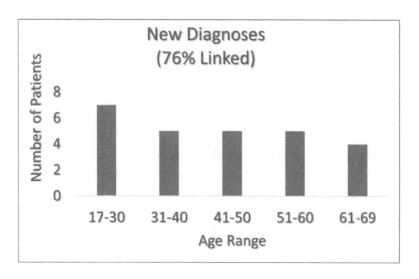

HOW TO TEACH ABOUT HARM REDUCTION

As with Chapter 9 and Chapter 11, this chapter is best taught by merging the evidence-based clinical guidelines with the health equity theme. Below is a list of topics from this chapter on which you can provide basic instruction. If your audience includes non-clinical administrators, then you can provide a cursory review of the guidelines and spend more time focusing on the potential stigma associated with drug use, HIV infection, etc. (Even if your audience is 100 percent clinical, this discussion of stigma is still important.)

- The CDC, USPSTF, AASLD, and IDSA age-based guidelines for HIV and HCV screening
- The importance of opt-out testing and getting rid of separate consent forms for HIV testing
- The benefits of early initiation of antiviral therapy for HIV and HCV infection
- The ASAM guidelines for the treatment of OUD (for residency programs, consider buprenorphine waiver training as a routine component of your curriculum)

See the additional reference in Notes for a discussion about ways to provide DAA therapy for uninsured patients at a dramatically reduced price.

CHAPTER 14

CONCLUSIONS ON HEALTH EQUITY

If you were hoping to hear one final bungle before this book ends, I am sorry to disappoint you by letting you know that the bungles ended with lucky Chapter 13. My monthly gaffes that I have confessed to before my medical students, resident physicians, audience participants, and colleagues for the past few years—and that I have shared with you in this book—are a reminder that none of us are perfect.

That is *Conclusion #1: No one is immune to the biases and missteps that are presented in this book, even if you are a member of the associated target group or a so-called expert.*

These were real events that happened to me (with minor details altered to preserve the privacy of those involved), some of which occurred after I began traveling around the country to lecture about and consult on how to achieve health equity. If anyone ever tries to make you feel shame when you are found to have a bias, or when you inadvertently use insensitive language, or when you lack awareness of a social problem, beware of that person—hypocrisy is lurking not far behind.

Once you accept that we all have biases, some of them unconscious or implicit, then the next step is to continue working to shed any tendencies to defend yourself when these biases are mentioned. It is normal to want to be perceived as a good person—and I would like to think that most of us are good people—but assuming a defensive posture is a hurdle on the path to achieving health equity.

Conclusion #2: Do not get defensive, but rather open your ears and your heart when you receive feedback about your potential role in perpetuating biases.

If you are busy trying to explain why you did not mean any harm, or that you were misunderstood, then you will not be able to clearly hear the point of view of the person engaging you. Also, for historically excluded or marginalized groups, it can be extremely frustrating when someone argues back while they are telling that person about their lived experience. It does not matter if you are friends with, married to, or have relatives in the target group being discussed, just stop and listen. I intend to do the same if I receive any constructive criticism about this book. After all, I am always on the lookout for new "bungles of the month" so that I can correct any behaviors that need to be addressed. (Feel free to share your own bungles with me via the "Contact Us" page at http://www.DoctorBonzo.com.)

Although the first two conclusions discuss individual behaviors, remember ***Conclusion #3***: *We should hold individuals accountable, but system changes are the most effective way to eliminate health inequities.*

In Chapter 3, we discussed how biases against pregnant and postpartum Black women lead to increased perinatal deaths, but statewide systemic changes in California were correlated with a 50 percent reduction in Black women's maternal mortality in just a few years. Similarly, to improve the poor rates of cervical cancer screening described in Chapter 6 among lesbian women and transgender men, you should not only educate physicians and health care providers about the problem, but you might need to implement protocols or install changes to your outpatient system. This could include improving nursing triage processes or using information technology to enhance your electronic medical record's ability to prompt clinicians to order appropriate screening tests.

Implicit bias trainings are some of the most popular health equity interventions that I am asked to provide, but this is only a beginning step. Instead of being reactionary to the biases that we uncover, our system must become one that overpowers both personal and institutional barriers.

As we continue to focus less on blaming individuals and more on removing systemic biases from healthcare organizations and structures, we should use the same large-scale approach outside of our hospital and clinic walls. A population health approach is more effective and more efficient than an individual approach to promoting health.

That leads to ***Conclusion #4***: *Community engagement and identification of local and regional partners are critical in achieving health equity.*

The average clinician or hospital executive might not have the available time or the knowledge about how to address issues such as housing or food insecurity, but there are usually advocacy organizations and local activists fighting for equity in these matters in most communities. There are also many public health and allied health professionals who experience territorial behavior from physicians despite providing services that their patients would benefit from. Engaging politicians and policymakers is one additional behavior that is not taught in many health professions schools, but it is necessary to facilitate moving beyond temporary fixes towards permanent solutions.

We should continue to look at how non-biomedical factors affect the morbidity and mortality of populations, and we should *normalize addressing the social determinants of health as a form of medical treatment—Conclusion #5*.

We outlined in Chapter 9 how social factors have a much larger influence on health outcomes than clinical care; throughout this book we have also discussed how people are often predisposed to certain health behaviors based on the social environments that they were raised in. Understanding these concepts will prevent judgmental attitudes towards patients for behaviors that increase the risk of disease or injury; it will also allow health care professionals and educators to focus on the interventions that will be the most effective and that will have the most long-lasting effects.

We will not realistically achieve health equity as a society until we view providing clean needles and syringes to people who inject drugs in the same way that we view administering a vaccine—after all, as we learned in the previous chapter, both actions are excellent at preventing viral and bacterial infections. I dream of the day when I can write a prescription for housing for an undomiciled person in the same way that I can write them a prescription for an antibiotic.

Conclusion #6: This book is by no means intended to be a comprehensive review of every existing health inequity in society; any chapter alone could have been an entire book by itself, and there are target groups that we did not discuss but who experience significant health disparities.

The topics and themes included in this book are the ones that I have been most commonly asked to speak about, and they are also the ones that I have encountered the most in my personal and professional life. Someone may be reading this book now and thinking, "I can't believe he didn't talk about (insert topic here)." This book presents a framework for addressing health disparities that can be applied to most situations of systemic and institutional bias, as well as to situations of personal bias and discrimination. Please remember that just because something was not included in this book does not mean it is not important. There will be regional and community-specific differences or variations that will make certain chapters more pressing than others, depending on the reader.

By this point of the book, you have heard me discuss the concept of *intersectionality* ad nauseum, so it might not surprise you that it is the focus of the final conclusion of this book.

Conclusion #7: *Although this book is presented in separate chapters, the lived experience of any patient, client, or other person that you meet is going to be composed of a confluence of elements from all of the chapters.*

A person's race, gender, weight, disability status, religion, sexual orientation, geographic location, and socioeconomic situation (especially their housing status!), will all interface with elements of society to impact that person's health and well-being. The way that these elements come together is going to be unique for each individual, so you cannot make assumptions about someone based on the experience of another person with similar demographics. That is why we dedicated an entire chapter (Chapter 8) to the importance of being culturally competent while also maintaining cultural humility. As you learn more about the target groups that we have discussed in this book, remember that each member of that group is not the same, and treat each person like an individual.

I hope that this book has been useful either as an introduction to health disparities, as a text to assist you in teaching about health inequities, or as a tool to help your organization develop a framework for achieving health equity. While I have included a lot of my personal experiences, I have made every effort to display the evidence that these concepts are based on along with successful examples that organizations have utilized. My use of humor (or at least my attempts at it) and self-deprecating anecdotes hopefully removed some of the anxiety, defensiveness, and confrontational reactions that so often accompany the provocative topics contained herein. If they were unsuccessful in doing so, then that is not necessarily a problem.

Health inequities lead to death and disability for millions of people, so it is not surprising that discussing them might provoke some strong emotions and discomfort. I do not generally find it useful to shame people, but we as a society should be ashamed for allowing certain behaviors to persist. For example, Chapter 9 outlined how we allow homelessness to continue despite the fact that it is more cost effective and has substantial health benefits when we provide housing for people. If you are uneasy when considering this, then I think that makes you a normal human being. This book is meant to accomplish something that has helped me tremendously in my health equity journey—helping people to become comfortable being uncomfortable.

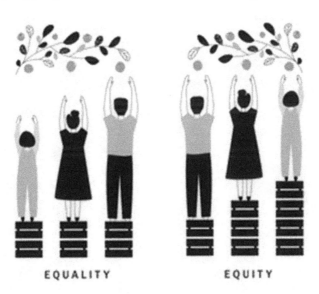

EQUALITY   EQUITY

Wishing you peace and love,
Dr. Bonzo

ACKNOWLEDGEMENTS

I am always hesitant to give acknowledgements because of a fear that I am going to forget someone. Therefore, I'll keep it brief and general; if I forget anyone, please charge it to my head and not to my heart.

First and foremost, I want to thank the Creator who fearfully and wonderfully made us all equal so that we are all deserving of an opportunity to achieve health equity. Thank you to my family, especially my wife Keisha and my three children, for your patience over the course of the year that it took me to write this book. Thank you to my parents, siblings, and extended family for always supporting my dreams.

Thanks to all the people who have participated in my education: from grade school, to college, to medical school, to residency, and finally to graduate school. Thanks to all my employers, past and present, for the opportunity to grow professionally. Thank you to all my patients—again, past and present—for the honor of being able to care for you. I appreciate you more than you'll ever know. Similarly, thanks to the medical students and resident physicians that I have been fortunate to teach and work with. You might not know it, but I also learned a lot from you.

I can't end without thanking Tieshena Davis, Pavita Singh, and the entire team at Publish Your Gift® for their patience and guidance during the publishing process. Tie, thank you for believing in me and in this project from day one, and thanks to IngramSpark for distributing my work.

Finally, I want to extend thanks to Dr. Jarret Patton for talking me into writing this book, and thanks to everyone who read this book. I hope that it lived up to your expectations, and I humbly await your feedback. I wish you all peace and blessings.

Sincerely,
Dr. Bonzo

NOTES

Preface

1. Andrews M. NBA unveils Black Lives Matter on Orlando court. NBA unveils Black Lives Matter on Orlando court (espn.com). *ESPN*; July 21, 2020 (last accessed December 22, 2020).

1. Alcendor DJ. Racial disparities-associated COVID-19 mortality among minority populations in the US. *J Clin Med* 2020; 9(8): 2442.

2. Coughlin SS, Moore JX, George V, Johnson JA, Hobbs J. COVID-19 among African Americans: From preliminary epidemiological surveillance data to public health action. *Am J Public Health* 2020; 110(8): 1157-1159.

3. Smedley BD, Stith AY, Nelson AR (eds). Unequal treatment: Confronting racial and ethnic disparities in healthcare. Washington, DC: National Academy Press, 2002.

4. C-SPAN. Dr. Anthony Fauci on health disparities in African American community. April 7, 2020; https://cs.pn/2wjp92O or https://www.youtube.com/watch?v=Q8eDzI4MiYQ (last accessed December 22, 2020).

5. Kohn LT, Corrigan JM, Donaldson MS (eds). Institute of Medicine (US) Committee on quality of health care in America. To err is human: Building a Safer Health System. Washington, DC: National Academies Press (US); 2000.

Footnote ξ: Terminology used to describe Latin American people: The terms Hispanic, Latino, Latina, and Latinx are often used interchangeably as a way to describe people from Latin America, although there is not uniformity or complete agreement about which terms are appropriate and in which settings they should be used.

- *"Hispanic" has traditionally been specific to people who speak Spanish and has been used to refer to people from Latin America or from Spain. It has fallen out of favor by some who would prefer that Latin American people be described independent of Spain given the history of colonialism in those countries.*

- *"Latino" has been used as a replacement for the term "Hispanic" that does not include people from Spain but does include people from some non-Spanish-speaking countries such as Brazil. The term Latino also includes reference to a Latin American man specifically, while Latina typically refers to a Latin American woman; in groups that include men and women, the default in the Spanish language is traditionally to use Latino (or Latinos if plural). Latinas typically refers to a group of Latin American women when no men are included in the group.*

- *"Latinx" has recently been introduced as an alternative to Latino/Latina that is more inclusive of people who have a non-binary gender identity (see Chapter 6 for more specifics about gender identity). Latinx is a term that is mostly used in the United States or in academia, and it is not commonly used in Latin American countries. The term has been criticized by some native Spanish speakers as it is difficult to pronounce in a language that does not include the letter "X" at the end of words. For this reason, some of these critics prefer the term Latine. There is also concern from some that insisting on using the term Latinx is an example of imperialistic behavior by some Americans attempting to "fix" the language of Hispanic/Latino communities.*

1. Introduction to Health Equity and Health Disparities

1. Braveman P. What are health disparities and health equity? We need to be clear. *Public Health Rep* 2014; 129 (Suppl 2): 5-8.

2. Healthy People 2020 (Department of Health and Human Services). Disparities; Disparities | Healthy People 2020 (last accessed October 29, 2021).

3. Crenshaw K. Demarginalizing the intersection of race and sex: A Black feminist critique of antidiscrimination doctrine, feminist theory and antiracist politics. *University of Chicago Legal Forum* Vol. 1989; Issue 1: Article 8.

4. U.S. Department of Health and Human Services. The Secretary's Advisory Committee on National Health Promotion and Disease Prevention Objectives for 2020. Phase I report: *Recommendations for the framework and format of Healthy People 2020*; Phase I report (healthypeople.gov) (last accessed October 29, 2021).

5. Smedley BD, Stith AY, Nelson AR (eds). Unequal treatment: Confronting racial and ethnic disparities in healthcare. Washington, DC: National Academy Press, 2002.

6. Baciu A, Negussie Y, Geller A, Weinstein JN (eds). National Academies of Sciences, Engineering, and Medicine; Health and Medicine Division; Board on Population Health and Public Health Practice; Committee on Community-Based Solutions to Promote Health Equity in the United

States. Communities in Action: Pathways to Health Equity. Chapter 2; The State of Health Disparities in the United States. Washington, DC: National Academies Press, 2017.

§*Footnote #2: Terminology used to describe sex and gender:*

- *In the overview of health disparities, the term "women" specifically refers to people assigned the sex of female at birth, and "men" refers to people assigned the sex of male at birth. Health statistics are often collected in this manner, so data on transgender people is often limited; this terminology is not used to purposefully exclude them or miscategorize them.*

- *Sex will be used in this way throughout this book, while gender may refer to several things, such as gender identity or gender expression.*

- *I will try to consistently clarify whether I am referring to sex, gender, gender identity, etc., with the use of the terms "men" and "women." If this is at all confusing, Chapter 6 should clarify things.*

2. Implicit (Unconscious) Bias

1. Association of American Medical Colleges (AAMC). Altering the course: Black men in medicine. 2015.

2. Talbert-Johnson C. Structural inequities and the achievement gap in urban schools. *Educ Urban Soc* 2004; 37(1): 22-36.

3. American Academy of Pediatrics (AAP) Council on Communications and Media (Hill D, Ameenuddin N, Chassiakos YR, et al.). Media and young minds. *Pediatrics* 2016; 138(5): e20162591.

4. American Academy of Pediatrics (AAP) Council on Communications and Media (Hill D, Ameenuddin N, Chassiakos YR, et al.). Media use in school-aged children and adolescents. *Pediatrics* 2016; 138(5): e20162591.

5. Ansell DA, McDonald EK. Bias, Black lives, and academic medicine. *NEJM* 2015; 372(12): 1087-1089.

6. Smedley BD, Stith AY, Nelson AR (eds). Unequal treatment: Confronting racial and ethnic disparities in healthcare. Washington, DC: National Academy Press, 2002.

7. Stuber J, Meyer I, Link B. Stigma, prejudice, discrimination and health. *Soc Sci Med* 2008; 67(3): 351-357.

8. Blair IV, Steiner JF, Fairclough DL, et al. Clinicians' implicit ethnic/racial bias and perceptions of care among Black and Latino patients. *Annals of Family Medicine* 2013; 11(1): 43-52.

9. Peckham C. Bias and burnout: Evil twins. http://www.medscape.com/viewarticle/85681 (last accessed January 18, 2021).

10. Berwick DM, Nolan TW, Whittington J. The triple aim: Care, health, and cost. *Health Affairs* 2008; 27(3): 759-769.

11. Mery G, Majumder S, Brown A, Dobrow MJ. What do we mean when we talk about the Triple Aim? A systematic review of evolving definitions and adaptations of the framework at the health system level. *Health Policy* 2017; 121(6): 629-636.

12. Schulman KA, Berlin JA, Harless W, et al. The effect of race and sex on physicians' recommendations for cardiac catheterization. *NEJM* 1999; 340(14): 618-626.

13. Abreu JM. Conscious and nonconscious African American stereotypes: Impact on first impression and diagnostic ratings by therapists. *Journal of Consulting and Clinical Psychology* 1999; 67(3): 387-393.

14. Borkhoff CM, Hawker GA, Kreder HJ, Glazier RH, Mahomed NN, Wright JG. The effect of patients' sex on physicians' recommendations for total knee arthroplasty. *CMAJ* 2008; 178(6): 681–687.

15. Chapman EN, Kaatz A, Carnes M. Physicians and implicit bias: How doctors may unwittingly perpetuate health care disparities. *J Gen Intern Med* 2013; 28(11): 1504-1510.

16. Van Ryn M, Burke J. The effect of race and socio-economic status on physicians' perceptions of patients. *Soc Sci Med* 2000; 50(6): 813-828.

17. Samet JM. Tobacco smoking: The leading cause of preventable disease worldwide. *Thorac Surg Clin* 2013; 23(2): 103-112.

18. Prochaska JO, Velicer WF. The transtheoretical model of health behavior change. *Am J Health Promot* 1997; 12(1): 38-48.

19. Capers Q. How Ohio State reduces implicit bias in admissions. https://www.youtube.com/watch?v=-053AUVYPw8 (last accessed August 4, 2020).

20. Greaney ML, Puleo E, Sprunck-Harrild K, Haines J, Houghton SC, Emmons KM. Social support for changing multiple behaviors: Factors associated with seeking support and the impact of offered support. *Health Educ Behav* 2018; 45(2): 198-206.

21. FitzGerald C, Hurst S. Implicit bias in healthcare professionals: A systematic review. *BMC Med Ethics* 2017; 18(1): 19.

22. Bauer S, Associated Press. Wisconsin's richest woman: 3 years with no state income tax. *TMJ4 News;* WI's richest woman paid no income tax for years (tmj4.com) (last accessed June 30, 2020).

3. Explicit Bias and Racism

1. Fugh-Berman A, Ahari S. Following the script: How drug reps make friends and influence doctors. *PLoS Med* 2007; 4(4): e150.

2. Applequist J, Ball JG. An updated analysis of direct-to-consumer television advertisements for prescription drugs. *Ann Fam Med* 2018; 16(3): 211-216.

3. Gilbody S, Wilson P, Watt I. Benefits and harms of direct to consumer advertising: A systematic review. *Qual Saf Health Care* 2005; 14(4): 246-250.

4. Ansell DA, McDonald EK. Bias, Black lives, and academic medicine. *NEJM* 2015; 372(12): 1087-1089.

5. Smedley BD, Stith AY, Nelson AR (eds). Unequal treatment: Confronting racial and ethnic disparities in healthcare. Washington, DC: National Academy Press, 2002.

6. Stuber J, Meyer I, Link B. Stigma, prejudice, discrimination and health. *Soc Sci Med* 2008; 67(3): 351-357.

7. Jones CP. Confronting Institutionalized Racism. *Phylon* 2003; 50(1-2): 7-22.

8. Elfrink T. "We are just gonna go out and start slaughtering them": Three cops fired after racist talk of killing black residents. *The Washington Post* - June 25, 2020; https://www.washingtonpost.com/nation/2020/06/25/wilmington-racist-police-recording/ (last accessed May 7, 2021).

9. Harrison LE, White BAA, McIntosh D. Explicit bias among fourth-year medical students. *Proc (Bayl Univ Med Cent)* 2019; 32(1): 50-53.

10. Carey TS, Garrett JM. The relation of race to outcomes and the use of health care services for acute low back pain. *Spine* 2003; 28: 390-394.

11. Chen I, Jurz J, Pasanen M, et al. Racial differences in opioid use for chronic nonmalignant pain. *J Gen Intern Med* 2005; 20: 593-598.

12. Goyal MK, Chamberlain JM, Johnson TJ, et al. Racial and ethnic differences in the management of pain among children diagnosed with

long bone fractures in pediatric emergency departments. *Pediatrics* 2020 May; 145: e20193370. Summary can be seen at https://childrensnational. org/news-and-events/childrens-newsroom/2018/racial-and-ethnic-differences-in-emergency-pain-relief-for-kids-with-broken-bones (last accessed September 30, 2020).

13. Goyal MK, Kuppermann N, Cleary SD, Teach SJ, Chamberlain JM. Racial disparities in pain management of children with appendicitis in emergency departments. *JAMA Pediatr* 2015; 169(11): 996-1002.

1. Welty LJ, Harrison AJ, Abram KM, et al. Health disparities in drug- and alcohol-use disorders: A 12-year longitudinal study of youths after detention. *Am J Public Health* 2016; 106(5): 872-880.

1. Scheralternet R. A racist stereotype is shattered: Study finds white youth are more likely to abuse hard drugs than black youth. *Salon* – April 6, 2016; A racist stereotype is shattered: Study finds white youth are more likely to abuse hard drugs than black youth | Salon.com (last accessed November 13, 2021).

2. Baudry E, Gusman N, Strang V, Thomas K, Villarreal E (Yale Global Health Justice Partnership). When the state fails: Maternal mortality & racial disparity in Georgia. 2017.

3. Warren K. As maternal mortality rises in the U.S., California bucks the trend. *Cronkite News* – December 16, 2019; California works to reverse high maternal mortality rates (azpbs.org) (last accessed May 4, 2020).

4. California Maternal Quality Care Collaborative. CA-PAMR (Maternal Mortality Review). CA-PAMR (Maternal Mortality Review) | California Maternal Quality Care Collaborative (cmqcc.org) (last accessed November 11, 2021).

5. Joynt J. Maternity care in California: A bundle of data. California Health Care Foundation - November 2019; Maternity Care in California, 2019: A Bundle of Data (chcf.org) (last accessed November 11, 2021).

6. Saluja B, Bryant Z. How implicit bias contributes to racial disparities in maternal morbidity and mortality in the United States. *J Womens Health (Larchmt)* 2021; 30(2): 270-273.

7. Russel S. Eradicating racism from maternity care begins with addressing implicit bias. *Nurs Womens Health* 2021; 25(3): 167-169.

8. Omeish Y, Kiernan S. Targeting bias to improve maternal care and outcomes for Black women in the USA. *EClinicalMedicine* 2020; 27: 100568.

9. Williams DR, Lawrence JA, Davis BA. Racism and health: Evidence and needed research. *Annu Rev Public Health* 2019; 40: 105-125.

10. Williams DR. How racism makes us sick. *TEDMED* 2016; https://www.ted.com/talks/david_r_williams_how_racism_makes_us_sick?language=en (last accessed May 4, 2020).

11. Krieger N, Rowley DL, Herman AA, Avery Byllye A, Phillips MT. Racism, sexism, and social class: implications for studies of health, disease, and well-being. *Am J Prev Med* 1993; 9(6 Suppl): 82-122.

12. Samuels A. *U.Va. report: Med students believe black people feel less pain than whites.* USA Today – April 5, 1016; http://college.usatoday.com/2016/04/05/uva-report-med-students-black-people-feel-less-pain/ (last accessed August 12, 2016).

13. Brooks KC. A silent curriculum. *JAMA* 2015; 313(19): 1909-1910.

14. Acosta DA. Achieving excellence through equity, diversity, and inclusion. *AAMC Insights* – January 14, 2020; Achieving excellence through equity, diversity, and inclusion | AAMC (last accessed May 6, 2021).

15. Coleman AL, Lipper KE, Taylor TE, Palmer SR, Education Counsel LLC (AAMC). Roadmap to diversity and educational excellence: Key legal and educational policy foundations for medical schools. Second ed (2014).

16. Trent M, Dooley DG, Douge' J, AAP Section on Adolescent Health, Council on Community Pediatrics, Committee on Adolescence. The impact of racism on child and adolescent health. *Pediatrics* 2019; 144(2): e20191765.

17. Folkenflik D. NPR ends Williams' contract after Muslim remarks. *NPR/GPB* – October 21, 2010; NPR ends Juan Williams' contract after Muslim remarks: NPR (last accessed October 7, 2020).

18. David Pakman Show. Juan Williams fired by NPR for these comments about Muslims. YouTube – October 21, 2010; Juan Williams fired by NPR for these comments about Muslims - YouTube (last accessed October 7, 2020).

19. Sun Journal (video captured by Lake Region Television). Gov. Paul LePage on Maine's drug problem. YouTube – January 7, 2016; https://www.youtube.com/watch?v=Jw_OxNkBbkQ (last accessed June 23, 2020).

20. Sharp D. Stats on drug trafficking, race don't back up Maine governor. *AP News* – September 5, 2016; https://apnews.

HEALTH EQUITY

com/3c501232c9e14fcfb0fe65267a1c34a0/Stats-on-drug-trafficking,-
race-donpercent27t-back-up-Maine-governor (last accessed June 23,
2020).

21. Mistler S. LePage: Mainers who carry concealed weapons could help rid
state of drug dealers. *Portland Press Herald* – January 28, 2016; LePage:
Mainers who carry concealed weapons could help rid state of drug dealers - CentralMaine.com (last accessed June 23, 2020).

22. Mistler S. LePage reiterates plan to use National Guard in drug epidem-
ic 'if necessary.' *Portland Press Herald* – August 11, 2015; https://www.
centralmaine.com/2015/08/11/lepage-reiterates-plan-to-use-nation-
al-guard-in-drug-epidemic-if-necessary/ (last accessed June 23, 2020).

[£]Footnote #3: References for internet search on recent mass shooters:

- *Since I described reviewing a minimum of ten results for several mass
shootings, I did not list the specific search results among the references
for this chapter. I chose not to list the more than forty results because
there was minimal content from these searches utilized in the text, with
the exception of the words "terrorist" and "Islamic terrorism" being used.*

- *Internet searches change from moment to moment, so the results of the
exercise described in this section will be different by the time of publication. For this particular search, I used the internet search engine Google.*

- *If you find results that differ significantly from the ones described herein,
please feel free to contact me via my website, www.DoctorBonzo.com.*

4. Race-Based Medical Decision-Making

1. Anderson MR, Moscou S, Fulchon C, Neuspiel DR. The role of race in
the clinical presentation. *Fam Med* 2001; 33(6): 430-434.

2. Douglas MD, Willock RJ, Respress E, et al. Applying a health equity lens
to evaluate and inform policy. *Ethn Dis* 2019; 29(Supp 2): 329-342.

3. Byyny RL. The social determinants of health. *The Pharos* 2012; Autumn:
2-7.

4. Satcher D. Include a social determinants of health approach to reduce
inequities. *Public Health Reports* 2010; 125(4): 6-7.

5. United States Census Bureau. Available from: https://www.census.gov/
topics/population/race/about.html (last accessed November 24, 2020).

6. Office of Management and the Budget. Revisions to the standard for the classification of federal data on race and ethnicity. *Federal Register* 1997; 62: 58781-90.

7. Hahn RA. The state of federal health statistics on racial and ethnic groups. *JAMA* 1992; 267(2): 268-71.

8. Graves, Jr. JL. The race myth: Why we pretend race exists in America: Plume 2004.

9. James PA, Oparil SO, Carter BL, Cushman WC, Dennison-Himmelfarb C, Handler J, et al. 2014 Evidence-Based guidelines for the management of high blood pressure in adults: Report from the panel members appointed to the eighth Joint National Committee (JNC 8). *JAMA* 2014; 311(5): 507-20.

10. ALLHAT Officers and Coordinators for the ALLHAT Collaborative Research Group. Major outcomes in high-risk hypertensive patients randomized to angiotensin-converting enzyme inhibitor or calcium channel blocker vs diuretic: The Antihypertensive and Lipid-Lowering Treatment to Prevent Heart Attack Trial (ALLHAT). *JAMA* 2002; 288(23): 2981-97.

11. Hellmer A, Slater N, Smithgall S. A review of ACE inhibitors and ARBs in Black patients with hypertension. *Ann Pharmacother* 2018; 52(11): 1143-51.

12. Smith DK, Lennon RP, Carlsgaard PB. Managing hypertension using combination therapy. *Am Fam Physician* 2020; 101(6): 341-9.

13. Flack JM, Sica DA, Barkis G, et al. Management of high blood pressure in blacks: An update of the International Society on Hypertension in Blacks consensus statement. *Hypertension* 2010; 56: 780-800.

14. Gallagher D, Visser M, De Meersman RE, et al. Appendicular skeletal muscle mass: Effects of age, gender, and ethnicity. *J Appl Physiol (1985)*. 1997; 83(1): 229-39.

15. Barondess DA, Nelson DA, Schlaen SE. Whole body bone, fat, and lean mass in black and white men. *J Bone Miner Res.* 1997; 12(6): 967-71.

16. Hsu J, Johansen KL, Hsu CY, Kaysen GA, Chertow GM. Higher serum creatinine concentrations in black patients with chronic kidney disease: Beyond nutritional status and body composition. *Clin J Am Soc Nephrol.* 2008; 3(4): 992-99.

17. Peralta CA, Lin F, Shlipak MG, et al. Race differences in prevalence of chronic kidney disease among young adults using creatinine-based

glomerular filtration rate-estimating equations. *Nephrol Dial Transplant* 2010; 25: 3934-9.

18. Vyas DA, Jones DS, Meadows AR, Diouf K, Nour NM, Schantz-Dunn J. Challenging the use of race in the vaginal birth after cesarean section calculator. *Women's Health Issues* 2019; 29(3): 201-204.

19. Lewiecki E, Wright N, Singer A. Racial disparities, FRAX, and the care of patients with osteoporosis. *Osteoporosis Int* 2020; 31(11): 2069-71.

20. Braun L. Race, ethnicity and lung function: A brief history. *Can J Respir Ther* 2015; 51(4): 99-101.

21. Braun L, Wolfgang M, Dickersin K. Defining race/ethnicity and explaining difference in research studies on lung function. *European Respiratory Journal* 2013; 41: 1362-70.

22. Braun L. Race correction and spirometry: Why history matters. *Chest* 2021; 159(4): 1670-1675.

23. Roberts DE. Fatal invention: How science, politics, and big business re-create race in the twenty-first century. New York; New Press: 2011.

24. American Medical Association. New AMA policies recognize race as a social, not biological, construct. https://www.ama-assn.org/press-center/press-releases/new-ama-policies-recognize-race-social-not-biological-construct (last accessed December 22, 2020).

25. Reddick B. Fallacies and dangers of practicing race-based medicine. *Am Fam Physician* 2021; 104(2): 122-123.

26. Torre LA, Siegel RL, Ward EM, Jemal A. Global cancer incidence and mortality rates and trends—An update. *Cancer Epidemiol Biomarkers Prev* 25(1): 16-27.

5. Sexism in Medicine

1. Dixon R. The Billy Graham Rule's unintended consequences. *Outreach Magazine* – October 13, 2021; https://outreachmagazine.com/resources/books/christian-living-books/69362-the-billy-graham-rules-unintended-consequences.html (last accessed November 28, 2021).

2. Association of American Medical Colleges (AAMC). Altering the course: Black men in medicine. 2015.

3. Ansell DA, McDonald EK. Bias, Black lives, and academic medicine. *NEJM* 2015; 372(12): 1087-1089.

4. Smedley BD, Stith AY, Nelson AR (eds). Unequal treatment: Confronting racial and ethnic disparities in healthcare. Washington, DC: National Academy Press, 2002.

5. Kriger N, Rowley DL, Herman AA, Avery Byllye A, Phillips MT. Racism, sexism, and social class: Implications for studies of health, disease, and well-being. *Am J Prev Med* 1993; 9(6 Suppl): 82-122.

6. Jones CP. Confronting Institutionalized Racism. *Phylon* 2003; 50(1-2): 7-22.

7. Glick P, Fiske ST. An ambivalent alliance: Hostile and benevolent sexism as complementary justifications for gender inequality. *Am Psychol* 2001; 56(2): 109-118.

8. Centers for Disease Control and Prevention. CDC health disparities and inequalities report—United States, 2013. *MMWR* 2013; 62:1–189.

9. Baciu A, Negussie Y, Geller A, Weinstein JN (eds). National Academies of Sciences, Engineering, and Medicine; Health and Medicine Division; Board on Population Health and Public Health Practice; Committee on Community-Based Solutions to Promote Health Equity in the United States. Communities in action: Pathways to health equity. Chapter 2; The State of Health Disparities in the United States. Washington, DC: National Academies Press, 2017.

10. Hornbuckle LM, Amutah-Onukagha N, Bryan A, et al. Health disparities in women. *Clin Med Insights Women's Health* 2017; 10.

11. Crenshaw K. Demarginalizing the intersection of race and sex: A Black feminist critique of antidiscrimination doctrine, feminist theory and antiracist politics. *University of Chicago Legal Forum* Vol. 1989; Issue 1: Article 8.

12. Tiller J, Reynolds S. Human trafficking in the emergency department: Improving our response to a vulnerable population. *West J Emerg Med* 2020; 21(3): 549-554.

13. Braileanu M, Edney E, Azar S, et al. Radiology, sexual harassment, and the #MeToo movement. *Acad Radiol* 2020; 28(4): 564-571.

14. Jena AB, Olenski AR, Blumenthal DM. Sex differences in physician salary in US public medical schools. *JAMA Intern Med* 2016; 176(9): 1294-1304.

15. Whaley CM, Koo T, Arora VM, Ganguli I, Gross N, Jena AB. Female physicians earn an estimated $2 million less than male physicians over a simulated 40-year career. *Health Affairs* 2021; 40(12): 1856-1864.

16. Silver JK, Blauwet CA, Bhatnagar S, et al. Women physicians are underrepresented in recognition awards from the Association of Academic Physiatrists. *Am J Phys Med Rehab* 2018; 97(1): 34-40.

17. Table 4A: Distribution of Women M.D. Faculty by Department and Rank, 2014. American Academy of Medical Colleges. Available at: https://www.aamc.org/download/411788/data/2014_table4a.pdf Published 2014 (last accessed September 30, 2016).

18. Silver JK, Bank AM, Slocum CS, et al. Women physicians are underrepresented in American Academy of Neurology recognition awards. *Neurology* 2018; 91(7): e603-e614.

6. Sexual and Gender Minorities (LGBTQ+ Health Disparities)

1. Centers for Disease Control and Prevention (CDC). Rates of new HIV diagnoses in the US and dependent areas, 2018. https://www.cdc.gov/hiv/statistics/overview/geographicdistribution.html (last accessed May 20, 2020).

2. Centers for Disease Control and Prevention (CDC). Lifetime risk of HIV diagnosis. https://www.cdc.gov/nchhstp/newsroom/2016/croi-press-release-risk.html (last accessed April 15, 2018).

3. U.S. Public Health Service. Preexposure prophylaxis for the prevention of HIV infection in the United States—2014: A clinical practice guideline. https://www.cdc.gov/hiv/pdf/prepprovidersupplement2014.pdf (last accessed October 26, 2017).

4. Grant RM, Lama JR, Anderson PL, et al. Preexposure chemoprophylaxis for HIV prevention in men who have sex with men. *N Engl J Med* 2010; 363(27): 2587-2599.

5. Thomson KA, Baeten JM, Mugo NR, Bekker LG, Celum CL, Heffron R. Tenofovir-based oral PrEP prevents HIV infection among women. *Curr Opin HIV AIDS* 2016; 11(1): 18-26.

6. Fonner VA, Dalglish SL, Kennedy CE, et al. Effectiveness and safety of oral HIV preexposure prophylaxis for all populations. *AIDS* 2016; 30(12): 1973-1983.

7. Bass B, Nagy H. Cultural competence in the care of LGBTQ patients. 2021 Oct 9. In: StatPearls [Internet]. Treasure Island (FL): StatPearls Publishing; 2021 Jan–. PMID: 33085323.

8. Goldberg SK, Rothblum ED, Russell ST, Meyer IH. Exploring the Q in LGBTQ: Demographic characteristic and sexuality of Queer people in a U.S. representative sample of sexual minorities. *Psychol Sex Orientat Gend Divers* 2020; 7(1): 101-112.

9. National Institutes of Health (NIH) Office of Intramural Research. Sexual and Gender Minority Health Scientific Interest Group. https://oir.nih.gov/sigs/sexual-gender-minority-health-scientific-interest-group (last accessed June 16, 2021).

10. Mayer KH, Bradford JB, Makadon HJ, Stall R, Goldhammer H, Landers S. Sexual and gender minority health: What we know and what needs to be done. *Am J Public Health* 2008; 98(6): 989-995.

11. Baciu A, Negussie Y, Geller A, Weinstein JN (eds). National Academies of Sciences, Engineering, and Medicine; Health and Medicine Division; Board on Population Health and Public Health Practice; Committee on Community-Based Solutions to Promote Health Equity in the United States. Communities in Action: Pathways to Health Equity. Chapter 2; The State of Health Disparities in the United States. Washington, DC: National Academies Press, 2017.

12. Hafeez H, Zeshan M, Tahir MA, Jahan N, Naveed S. Health care disparities among lesbian, gay, bisexual, and transgender youth: A literature review. *Cureus* 2017; 9(4): e1184.

13. Pharr JR. Health disparities among lesbian, gay, bisexual, transgender, and nonbinary adults 50 years old and older in the United States. *LGBT Health* 2021; 8(7): 473-485.

14. Curry SJ, Krist AH, Owens DK, et al (US Preventive Services Task Force). Screening for cervical cancer: US Preventive Services Task Force recommendation statement. *JAMA* 2018; 320(7): 674-686.

15. Tracy JK, Schluterman NH, Greenberg DR. Understanding cervical cancer screening among lesbians: A national survey. *BMC Public Health* 2013; 13: 442.

16. Tracy JK, Lydecker AD, Ireland L. Barriers to cervical cancer screening among lesbians. *J Women's Health (Larchmt)* 2010; 19(2): 229-237.

17. Curmi C, Peters K, Salamonson Y. Barriers to cervical cancer screening experienced by lesbian women: A qualitative study. *Journal of Clinical Nursing* 2016; 25(23-24): 3643-3651.

18. Johnson MJ, Nemeth LS, Mueller M, Eliason MJ, Stuart GW. Qualitative study of cervical cancer screening among lesbian and bisexual women and transgender men. *Cancer Nurs* 2016; 39(6): 455-463.

19. Light A, Wang LF, Zeymo A, Gomez-Lobo V. Family planning and contraception use in transgender men. *Contraception* 2018; 98(4): 266-269.

20. Tervalon M, Murray-Garcia. Cultural humility versus cultural competence: A critical distinction in defining physician training outcomes in multicultural education. *J Health Care Poor Underserved* 1998; 9(2): 117-25.

21. Krempasky C, Harris M, Abern L, Grimstad F. Contraception across the transmasculine spectrum. *Am J Obstet Gynecol* 2020; 222(2): 134-143.

22. The World Professional Association for Transgender Health (WPATH). Standards of care for the health of transsexual, transgender, and gender nonconforming people. *Standards of Care (SOC), Version 7.*

23. Bonvicini KA. LGBT healthcare disparities: What progress have we made? *Patient Educ Couns* 2017; 100(12): 2357-2361.

24. Appiah KA. Should patients be allowed to choose—or refuse—doctors by race or gender? *New York Times Magazine* August 6, 2019. https://www.nytimes.com/2019/08/06/magazine/should-patients-be-allowed-to-choose-or-refuse-doctors-by-race-or-gender.html (last accessed September 23, 2019).

25. Coleman AL, Lipper KE, Taylor TE, Palmer SR, Education Counsel LLC (AAMC). Roadmap to diversity and educational excellence: Key legal and educational policy foundations for medical schools. Second ed (2014).

26. Przedworski JM, Dovidio JF, Hardeman RR, et al. A comparison of the mental health of and well-being of sexual minority and heterosexual first-year medical students: A report from the Medical Student CHANGE Study. *Acad Med* 2015; 90(5): 652-659.

27. Eckstrand KL, Sciolla AF. Implementing curricular and institutional climate changes to improve health care for individuals who are LGBT, gender nonconforming, or born with DSD. AAMC Executive Summary (2015).

7. Religious Tolerance

1. Appiah KA. Should patients be allowed to choose—or refuse—doctors by race or gender? *New York Times Magazine* August 6, 2019. https://www.nytimes.com/2019/08/06/magazine/should-patients-be-allowed-to-choose-or-refuse-doctors-by-race-or-gender.html (last accessed September 23, 2019).

2. Samari G, Alcalá HE, Sharif MZ. Islamophobia, health, and public health: A systematic literature review. *Am J Public Health* 2018; 108(6): e1-e9.

3. Khalife T, Pettit JM, Weiss BD. Caring for Muslim patients who fast during Ramadan. *Am Fam Physician* 2015; 91(9): 640-642.

4. Abolaban H, Al-Moujahed A. Muslim patients in Ramadan: A review for primary care physicians. *Avicenna J Med* 2017; 7(3): 81-87.

5. Padela AI, Raza A. American Muslim health disparities: The state of the Medline literature. *Journal of Health Disparities Research and Practice* 2015; 8(1): 1-9.

6. Nowakowski ACH, Sumerau JE. Health disparities in nonreligious and religious older adults in the United States: A descriptive epidemiology of 16 common chronic conditions. *Secularism and Nonreligion* 2017; 6(4): 1-15.

7. Paul-Emile K, Critchfield JM, Wheeler M, de Bourmont S, Fernandez A. Addressing patient bias toward health care workers: Recommendations for medical centers. *Ann Intern Med* 2020; 173(6): 468-473.

8. Warsame RM, Hayes SN. Mayo Clinic's 5-step policy for responding to bias incidents. *AMA Journal of Ethics* 2019; 21(6): E521-29.

9. Paul-Emile K, Smith AK, Lo B, Fernandez A. Dealing with racist patients. *N Engl J Med* 2016; 374(8): 708-711.

8. Cultural Competence Versus Cultural Humility

1. Bradford L, Goodman A. Cervical cancer screening and prevention in low-resource settings. *Clin Obstet Gynecol* 2013; 56(1): 76-87.

2. Pew Research Center. Religion in Latin America: Widespread change in a historically Catholic region. November 13, 2014.

3. Anderson LM, Scrimshaw SC, Fullilove MT, Fielding JE, Normand J (Task Force on Community Preventive Services). Culturally competent healthcare systems: A systematic review. *Am J Prev Med* 2003; 24(Suppl 3): 68-79.

4. Tervalon M, Murray-Garcia. Cultural humility versus cultural competence: A critical distinction in defining physician training outcomes in multicultural education. *J Health Care Poor Underserved* 1998; 9(2): 117-125.

5. Borkan JM, Culhane-Pera KA, Goldman RE. Towards cultural humility in healthcare for culturally diverse Rhode Island. *Med Health RI.* 2008; 91(12): 361-364.

6. Sanders MA, Akinlaja OA, Gass VR. Epidural anesthesia in the Latina population. *Obstetrics & Gynecology* 2015; 125: 28S-29S.

7. Hansen DA, Measom RJ, Scott B. Epidural analgesia in Hispanic parturients: A single-blinded prospective cohort study on the effects of an educational intervention on epidural analgesia utilization. *J Obstet Anaesth Crit Care* 2017; 7(2): 90-94.

8. Spanish-Speaking Hispanic women less likely to receive labor analgesia. Spanish-Speaking Hispanic women less likely to receive labor analgesia (newswise.com) (last accessed November 30, 2020).

9. Firger J. Circumcision rates declining in U.S., study says. Circumcision rates declining in U.S. infants, raising health risks later in life - CBS News (last accessed November 30, 2020).

10. American Academy of Pediatrics Task Force on Circumcision. Blank S, Brady M, Buerk E, et al. Male circumcision. *Pediatrics* 2012; 130(3): e756-e785.

11. Millet GA, Flores SA, Marks G, Reed JB, Herbst JH. Circumcision status and risk of HIV and sexually transmitted infections among men who have sex with men: a meta-analysis. *JAMA* 2008; 300(14): 1674-1684.

12. Cottrell LS. The competent community. Chapter 11 In: Kaplan BH, Wilson RN, Leighton AH (eds.). *Further Explorations in Social Psychiatry.* New York: Basic Books, 1976.

13. Kumar R, Bhattacharya S, Sharma N, Thiyagarajan A. Cultural competence in family practice and primary care settings. *J Family Med Prim Care* 2019; 8(1): 1-4.

14. Braddock CH, Crandall SJ, Gruppen LD, Nuñez AE, Price-Haywood EG (AAMC). Assessing change: Evaluating cultural competence education and training. (March 2015).

9. Social Determinants of Health and Homelessness

1. Byyny RL. The social determinants of health. *The Pharos* 2012; Autumn: 2-7.

2. Satcher D. Include a social determinants of health approach to reduce inequities. *Public Health Reports* 2010; 125(4): 6-7.

3. Los Angeles County Department of Public Health. Social determinants of health: How social and economic factors affect health. http://publichealth.lacounty.gov/epi/docs/SocialD_Final_Web.pdf (last accessed April 27, 2017).

4. Braun L. Race, ethnicity and lung function: A brief history. *Can J Respir Ther* 2015; 51(4): 99-101.

5. Braun L, Wolfgang M, Dickersin K. Defining race/ethnicity and explaining difference in research studies on lung function. *European Respiratory Journal* 2013; 41: 1362-1370.

6. Beck AF, Huang B, Chundur R, Kahn RS. Housing code violation density associated with emergency department and hospital use by children with asthma. *Health Aff*airs November 2014;33(11) 1993-2002.

7. Montauk SL. The homeless in America: Adapting your practice. *Am Fam Physician* 2006; 74(7): 1132-1138.

8. Tong MS, Kaplan LM, Guzman D, Ponath C, Kushel MB. Persistent homelessness and violent victimization among older adults in the HOPE HOME Study. *J Interpers Violence* 2021; 36(17-18): 8519-8537.

9. Downtown Emergency Service Center. Seven standards of housing first. https://www.desc.org/what-we-do/housing/housing-first/ (last accessed April 17, 2018).

10. Watson DP, Orwat J, Wagner DE, Shuman V, Tolliver R. The housing first model (HFM) fidelity index: Designing and testing a tool for measuring integrity of housing programs that serve active substance abusers. *Subst Abus Treat Prev Policy* 2013; 8: 1-16.

11. Perlman J, Parvensky J. Denver Housing First Collaborative: Cost benefit analysis and program outcomes report. 2006. https://shnny.org/uploads/Supportive_Housing_in_Denver.pdf (last accessed April 17, 2018).

12. Tsemberis S, Stefancic A. Housing First for long-term shelter dwellers with psychiatric disabilities in a suburban county: A four-year study of housing access and retention. *J Prim Prev* 2007; 28(3-4): 265-79.

13. Malinen F. Finland's 'Housing First' policy proves that homelessness is avoidable. *Equal Times;* Finland's 'Housing First' policy proves that homelessness is avoidable - Equal Times (last accessed January 28, 2021).

14. Goldfarb S. Take two aspirin and call me by my pronouns. *Wall Street Journal;* September 12, 2019 (last accessed December 15, 2021).

15. Flack JM, Sica DA, Barkis G, et al. Management of high blood pressure in blacks: An update of the International Society on Hypertension in Blacks consensus statement. *Hypertension* 2010; 56: 780-800.

10. Health Inequities Affecting Disabled/Differently Abled People

1. Fenell Z. Stop saying 'wheelchair-bound' and other outdated and offensive terms to people with disabilities. *Impact, Huffington Post;* November 11, 2013, updated November 12, 2015. https://www.huffingtonpost.com/2013/11/01/how-to-talk-to-person-with-disability_n_4191830.html (last accessed January 26, 2018).

2. Janz HL. Ableism: The undiagnosed malady afflicting medicine. *CMAJ* 2019; 191(17): E478-E479.

3. Neilson S. Ableism in the medical profession. *CMAJ* 2020; 192(15): E411-E412.

4. Campbell FK. Inciting legal fictions: Disability's date with ontology and the ableist body of the law. *Griffith Law Rev* 2001; 10: 42-62.

5. Baciu A, Negussie Y, Geller A, Weinstein JN (eds). National Academies of Sciences, Engineering, and Medicine; Health and Medicine Division; Board on Population Health and Public Health Practice; Committee on Community-Based Solutions to Promote Health Equity in the United States. Communities in Action: Pathways to Health Equity. Chapter 2; The State of Health Disparities in the United States. Washington, DC: National Academies Press, 2017.

6. Schwab W. (video captured by The American Board of Family Medicine). People with disabilities (Developmental and intellectual disabilities). YouTube – August 3, 2017; https://www.youtube.com/watch?v=x-Vx8d3ne9bw (last accessed January 28, 2021).

7. National Association of State Directors of Developmental Disability Services. http://www.nationalcoreindicators.org/upload/presentation/FINAL_NASDDDS_2014_Health_Disparities.pdf (last accessed January 28, 2021).

8. Havercamp SM, Scott HM. National health surveillance of adults with disabilities, adults with intellectual and developmental disabilities, and adults with no disabilities. *Disabil Health J* 2015; 8(2): 165-72.

9. Kattari SK. Ableist microaggressions and the mental health of disabled adults. *Community Ment Health J* 2020; 56(6): 1170-1179.

10. Conover KJ, Israel T. Microaggressions and social support among sexual minorities with physical disabilities. *Rehabil Psychol* 2019; 64(2): 167-178.

11. Academy of Developmental Medicine and Dentistry. Health disparities consensus statement. https://aadmd.org/articles/health-disparities-consensus-statement (last accessed January 28, 2021).

12. Grady A, Fiori A, Patel D, Nysenbaum J. Profile of Medicaid enrollees with sickle cell disease: A high need, high cost population. *PLoS One* 2021; 16(10): e0257796.

13. Lubeck D, Agodoa I, Bhakta N, et al. Estimated life expectancy and income of patients with sickle cell disease compared with those without sickle cell disease. *JAMA Netw Open* 2019; 2(11): e1915374.

14. National Heart, Lung, and Blood Institute (NHLBI), U.S. Department of Health and Human Services (National Institutes of Health). Evidence-based management of sickle cell disease: Expert Panel Report, 2014.

11. Patients Diagnosed with "Morbid Obesity"

1. Prochaska JO, Velicer WF. The transtheoretical model of health behavior change. *Am J Health Promot* 1997; 12(1): 38-48.

2. Centers for Disease Control and Prevention (CDC). Defining adult overweight & obesity. https://www.cdc.gov/obesity/adult/defining.html (page last reviewed June 7, 2021).

3. Puhl R, Brownell KD. Bias, discrimination, and obesity. *Obes Res* 2001; 9(12): 788-805.

4. Roehling MV. Weight-based discrimination in employment: Psychological and legal aspects. *Pers Psychol* 2006; 52(4): 969-1016.

5. Paul RJ, Townsend JB. Shape up or ship out? Employment discrimination against the overweight. *Empl Responsib Rights J* 1995; 8: 133-145.

6. Wharton S, Lau DCW, Vallis M, et al. Obesity in adults: A clinical practice guidelines. *CMAJ* 2020; 192(31): E875-E891.

7. Nuttall FQ. Body mass index: Obesity, BMI, and Health: A critical review. *Nutr Today* 2015; 50(3): 117-128.

8. Harp JB, Hecht L. Obesity in the National Football League. *JAMA* 2005; 293(9): 1061-1062.

9. Berwick DM, Nolan TW, Whittington J. The triple aim: Care, health, and cost. *Health Affairs* 2008; 27(3): 759-769.

10. Mery G, Majumder S, Brown A, Dobrow MJ. What do we mean when we talk about the Triple Aim? A systematic review of evolving definitions and adaptations of the framework at the health system level. *Health Policy* 2017; 121(6): 629-636.

11. Garvey WT, Mechanick JI, Brett EM, et al. (Reviewers of the AACE/ACE Obesity Clinical Practice Guidelines). American Association of Clinical Endocrinologists and American College of Endocrinology comprehensive clinical practice guidelines for medical care of patients with obesity. *Endocr Practice* 2016; 22(Suppl 3): 1-205.

12. Gonzalez-Campoy JM, St. Jeor ST, Castorino K, et al. Clinical Practice Guidelines for healthy eating for the prevention and treatment of metabolic and endocrine diseases in adults: Cosponsored by the American Association of Clinical Endocrinologists/The American College of Endocrinology and the Obesity Society. *Endocr Practice* 2013; 19(Suppl 3): 1-82.

12. Rural Health Disparities

1. Hart LG, Larson EH, Lishner DM. Rural definitions for health policy and research. *Am J Public Health* 2004; 95(7): 1149-1155.

2. Health Resources and Services Administration (HRSA). Defining rural population. U.S. Department of Health & Human Services Guidance Portal – published June 25, 2020; https://www.hhs.gov/guidance/document/defining-rural-population (last accessed August 31, 2021).

3. Wilger S. Definition of frontier. National Rural Health Association Policy Brief; approved February 2016 by the Rural Health Congress; https://www.ruralhealth.us/getattachment/Advocate/Policy-Documents/NRHAFrontierDefPolicyPaperFeb2016.pdf.aspx (last accessed August 31, 2021).

4. Baciu A, Negussie Y, Geller A, Weinstein JN (eds). National Academies of Sciences, Engineering, and Medicine; Health and Medicine Division; Board on Population Health and Public Health Practice; Committee on Community-Based Solutions to Promote Health Equity in the United

States. Communities in Action: Pathways to Health Equity. Chapter 2; The State of Health Disparities in the United States. Washington, DC: National Academies Press, 2017.

5. Monnat SM, Beeler Pickett C. Rural/urban differences in self-related health: Examining the roles of county size and metropolitan adjacency. *Health Place* 2011; 17(1): 311-319.

6. Bethea TN, Lopez RP, Cozier YC, White LF, McClean MD. The relationship between rural status, individual characteristics, and self-rated health in the Behavioral Risk Factor Surveillance System. *J Rural Health* 2012; 28(4): 327-328.

7. Matthews KA, Croft JB, Liu Y, et al. Health-related behaviors by urban-rural county classification: United States, 2013. *MMWR Surveill Summ* 2017; 66(5): 1-8.

8. Douthit N, Kiv S, Dwolatzky T, Biswas S. Exposing some important barriers to health care access in the rural USA. *Public Health* 2015; 129(6): 611-620.

9. Abrams LR, Myrsklyä M, Mehta NK. The growing rural-urban divide in US life expectancy: Contribution of cardiovascular disease and other major causes of death. *Int J Epidemiol* 2021; 50(6): 1970-1978.

10. Henley SJ, Anderson RN, Thomas CC, Massetti GM, Peaker B, Richardson LC. Invasive cancer incidence, 2004-2013, and deaths, 2006-2015, in nonmetropolitan and metropolitan counties – United States. *MMWR Surveill Summ* 2017; 66(14): 1-13.

11. Heron M. Deaths: Leading causes for 2019. *National Vital Statistics Reports* 2021; 70(9): 1-17.

12. Georgia Board for Physician Workforce. Georgia counties with no physicians. https://healthcareworkforce.georgia.gov/document/counties-without-primary-care-practitioners/download (last accessed March 30, 2021).

13. Ham N, Dekutowski SM, Edwards C. The Rural Hospital Stabilization Program: A comprehensive report. Georgia Department of Community Health – December 2019; https://dch.georgia.gov/document/document/ruralhospitalstabilizationcomprehensivereportcompresseddec2019pdf/download (last accessed March 30, 2021).

14. Mosley D, Debehnke D (Navigant). Rural hospital sustainability: New data show worsening situation for rural hospitals, residents. Navigant Consulting, Inc. – February 2019; https://cqrcengage.com/ancor/file/

X09PcoJsPrh/Navigant_Rural_Hospitals_Report_2019.pdf (last accessed March 30, 2021).

15. Ellison A. State-by-state breakdown of 134 rural hospital closures. *Beckers Hospital CFO Report* – November 24, 2020; https://www.beckershospitalreview.com/finance/state-by-state-breakdown-of-134-rural-hospital-closures.html (last accessed March 30, 2021).

16. Mohamoud YA, Kirby RS, Ehrenthal DB. County poverty, urban-rural classification, and the causes of term infant death: United States, 2012-2015. *Public Health Rep* 2021; 136(5): 584-594.

17. Ehrenthal DB, Kuo HD, Kirby RS. Infant mortality in rural and nonrural counties in the United States. *Pediatrics* 2020; 146(5): e20200464.

18. Paul R, Adeyemi O, Ghosh H, Han D. Progression of COVID-19 from urban to rural areas in the United States: A spatiotemporal analysis of prevalence rates. *J Rural Health* 2020; 36(4): 591-601.

19. Henning-Smith CE, Hernandez AM, Hardeman RR, Ramirez MR, Kozhimannil KB. Rural counties with majority Black or Indigenous populations suffer the highest rates of premature death in the US. *Health Aff* 2019; 38(12): 2019-2026.

20. Centers for Disease Control and Prevention (CDC). Preventing chronic diseases and promoting health in rural communities – last reviewed July 1, 2019; https://www.cdc.gov/chronicdisease/pdf/factsheets/Rural-Health-Overview-H.pdf (last accessed August 30, 2021).

21. Butzner M, Cuffee Y. Telehealth interventions and outcomes across rural communities in the United States: Narrative review. *J Med Internet Res* 2021; 23(8): e29575.

22. Boudreaux M, Barath D, Blewett LA. Recent changes in health insurance coverage for urban and rural veterans: Evidence from the first year of the Affordable Care Act. *Mil Med* 2019; 184(1-2): e76-e82.

23. Meurer LN, Young SA, Meurer JR, Johnson SL, Gilbert IA, Diehr S (Urban and Community Health Pathway Planning Council). The Urban and Community Health Pathway: Preparing socially responsive physicians through community-engaged learning. *Am J Prev Med* 2011; 41(4): S228-S236.

24. Goralnick E, Ezeibe C, Chaudhary MA, et al. Defining a research agenda for layperson prehospital hemorrhage control. *JAMA Netw Open* 2020; 3(7): e209393.

13 Harm Reduction and People Who Use Drugs

1. Schillie S, Wester C, Osborne M, Wesolowski L, Ryerson AB. CDC recommendations for hepatitis C screening among adults—United States, 2020. *MMWR Recomm Rep* 2020; 69(No. RR-2): 1-17.

2. American Association for the Study of Liver Diseases (AASLD), Infectious Diseases Society of America (IDSA). Recommendations for testing, managing, and treating hepatitis C. http://www.hcvguidelines.org/ (last updated November 6, 2019).

3. Chou R, Dana T, Fu R, et al. Screening for hepatitis C virus infection in adolescents and adults: A systematic review update for the U.S. Preventive Services Task Force. Evidence Synthesis No. 188. AHRQ Publication No. 19-05256-EF-1. Rockville, MD: Agency for Health Research and Quality; 2019.

4. U.S. Preventive Services Task Force (USPSTF). Hepatitis C virus infection in adults and adolescents: Screening. https://www.uspreventiveservicestaskforce.org/Page/Document/ draft-recommendation-statement/ hepatitis-c-screening (last updated September 23, 2019).

5. U.S. Preventive Services Task Force (USPSTF). Screening for HIV infection: US Preventive Services Task Force Recommendation Statement. *JAMA* 2019; 321(23): 2326-2336.

6. Branson BM, Handsfield HH, Lampe MA, et al. Revised recommendations for HIV testing of adults, adolescents, and pregnant women in health-care settings. *MMWR* 2006; 55(No. RR-14): 1-17.

7. Lok AS, Chung RT, Vargas HE, Kim AY, Naggie S, Powderly WG. Benefits of direct-acting antivirals for hepatitis C. *Ann Intern Med* 2017; 167(11): 812-813.

8. Kalidindi Y, Jung J, Feldman R, Riley III, T. Association of direct-acting antiviral treatment with mortality among Medicare beneficiaries with hepatitis C. *JAMA Netw Open* 2020; 3(7): e2011055.

9. Centers for Disease Control and Prevention. Hepatitis C FAQs for the public. https://www.cdc.gov/hepatitis/hcv/cfaq.htm (last updated July 28, 2020).

10. Centers for Disease Control and Prevention (CDC). Rates of new HIV diagnoses in the US and dependent areas, 2018. https://www.cdc.gov/hiv/statistics/overview/geographicdistribution.html (last accessed May 20, 2020).

11. Van Handel MM, Rose CE, Hallisley EJ, et al. County-level vulnerability assessment for rapid dissemination of HIV or HCV infections among persons who inject drugs, United States. *J Acquir Immune Defic Syndr* 2016; 73(3): 323-331.

12. Reddick B, O'Ree M. Improving access to hepatitis C treatment for uninsured patients in Southeast Georgia. *J Ga Public Health Assoc* 2020; 8(1): 11-13.

13. Des Jarlais DC, Nugent A, Solberg A, Feelemyer J, Mermin J, Holtzman D. Syringe service programs for persons who inject drugs in urban, suburban, and rural areas—United States, 2013. *MMWR* 2015; 64(48): 1337-41.

14. Aspinall EJ, Nambiar D, Goldberg DJ, et al. Are needle and syringe programmes associated with a reduction in HIV transmission among people who inject drugs? A systematic review and meta-analysis. *Int J Epidemiol* 2014; 43(1): 235-248.

15. Nguyen, TQ, Weir BW, Des Jarlais DC, Pinkerton SD, Holtgrave DT. Syringe exchange in the United States: A national level economic evaluation of hypothetical increases in investment. *AIDS and Behavior* 2014; 18(11): 2144-2155.

16. Hagan H, McGough JP, Thiede H, Hopkins S, Duchin J, Alexander ER. Reduced injection frequency and increased entry and retention in drug treatment associated with needle-exchange participation in Seattle drug injectors. *J Subst Abuse Treat* 2000; 19(3): 247-252.

17. Armbruster AL, Watford JB. HB 217 – Crimes and Offenses, 36 GA. ST. U. L. REV. 27. *Georgia State University Law Review* 2019; 36(1): 27-37 (Article 2).

18. Abdala N, Gleghorn A, Carney JM, Heimer R. Use of bleach to disinfect HIV-1 contaminated syringes. American Clinical Laboratory, 20(6): 26-28.

19. World Health Organization (WHO). Evidence for action on HIV/AIDS and injecting drug use technical paper and policy briefings: Effectiveness of sterile needle and syringe programming in reducing HIV/AIDS among injecting drug users. https://www.who.int/hiv/pub/prev_care/effectivenesssterileneedle.pdf; Geneva, 2004 (last accessed April 28, 2021).

20. American Society of Addiction Medicine. Definition of addiction. Adopted September 15, 2019; https://www.asam.org/docs/default-source/

quality-science/asam's-2019-definition-of-addiction-(1).pdf?s-fvrsn=b8b64fc2_2 (last accessed April 28, 2021).

21. Sussman S, Sussman AN. Considering the definition of addiction. *Int J Environ Res Public Health* 2011; 8(10): 4025-4038.

22. Lenton S, Single E. The definition of harm reduction. *Drug Alcohol Rev* 1998; 17(2): 213-219.

23. Single E. Defining harm reduction. *Drug Alcohol Rev* 1995; 14(3): 287-290.

24. Crotty K, Freedman KI, Kampman KM. Executive summary of the focused update of the ASAM National Practice Guideline for the treatment of opioid use disorder. *J Addict Med* 2020; 14(2): 99-112.

25. Barnett ML, Lee D, Frank RG. In rural areas, buprenorphine waiver adoption since 2017 driven by nurse practitioners and physician assistants. *Health Aff (Millwood)* 2019; 38(12): 2048-2056.

26. Stokes DC, Perrone J. Increasing short- and long-term buprenorphine treatment capacity: Providing waiver training for medical students. *Acad Med* 2022; 97(2): 182-187.

ABOUT THE AUTHOR

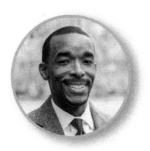

DR. BONZO REDDICK is a professor in the Community Medicine and Family Medicine departments at Mercer University School of Medicine. He previously served as the Associate Dean of Diversity, Equity & Inclusion. After receiving his bachelor's degree from Morehouse College and his medical degree from Morehouse School of Medicine, Dr. Bonzo attended University of North Carolina at Chapel Hill, where he completed a family medicine residency, two faculty development fellowships, and a Master of Public Health.

Dr. Bonzo has received sixteen teaching awards, was named Georgia Family Physician of the Year in 2021, and has served on the Health Equity Council for the Georgia Department of Public Health. A Fellow of the American Academy of Family Physicians, Dr. Bonzo provides mobile homeless care at a federally designated Healthcare for the Homeless site.

Dr. Bonzo lives in Savannah, Georgia, with his wife, three children, and dog.

Learn more at
www.DoctorBonzo.com

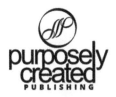

CREATING DISTINCTIVE BOOKS
WITH INTENTIONAL RESULTS

We're a collaborative group of creative masterminds
with a mission to produce high-quality books to position
you for monumental success in the marketplace.

Our professional team of writers, editors, designers,
and marketing strategists work closely together to ensure
that every detail of your book is a clear representation
of the message in your writing.

Want to know more?
Write to us at info@publishyourgift.com
or call (888) 949-6228

Discover great books, exclusive offers, and more at
www.PublishYourGift.com

Connect with us on social media

@publishyourgift

Printed in the USA
CPSIA information can be obtained
at www.ICGtesting.com
LVHW010720230124
768658LV00015B/906